REVERSE THE AGING PROCESS OF YOUR FACE

A SIMPLE TECHNIQUE THAT WORKS

To Barbara
Enjoy reading

RACHEL PERRY

Rachel P

D1534570

Avery Publishing Group
Garden City Park, New York

Cover designer: Bill Cuffari
Cover photographer: Harry Langdon
Typesetters: Bonnie Freid and William Gonzalez
Printer: Paragon Press, Honesdale, PA

Library of Congress Cataloging-In-Publication Data

Perry, Rachel (Rachel R.)
    Reverse the aging process of your face : a simple technique that
works / Rachel Perry.
        p.   cm.
    Includes bibliographical references and index.
    ISBN 0-89529-625-X (pbk.)
    1. Skin—Care and hygiene.   2. Skin—Aging.   I. Title.
RL87.P47 1995   95-18688
646.7'26—dc20   CIP

Printed in the United States of America.

10   9   8   7   6   5   4   3   2

CONTENTS

To Sheryl Carson, my beloved friend,
who inspired me all my life
to fulfill my creative potential.

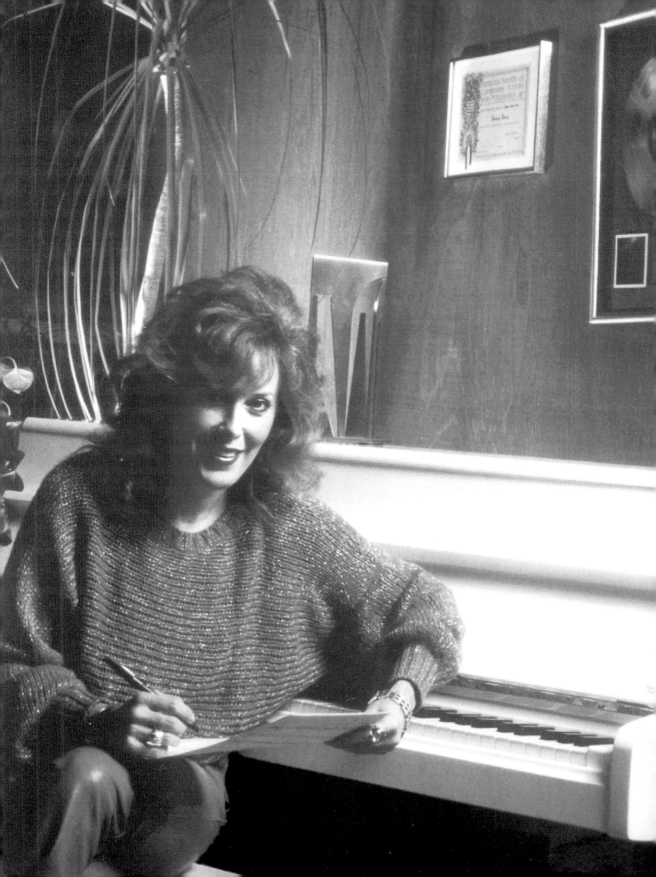

PREFACE

Like many women in our society, I grew up believing (erroneously) that growing older would mean losing my looks, my sex appeal, and my chances for a new career and success. It has taken me a long time to unlearn all of these falsehoods. In fact, as I get older, I am always continuing to learn that, contrary to my former beliefs, my looks keep improving, my sexuality is not disappearing, and I have more energy and creativity at my fingertips than ever. I am involved in doing things I love to do, and feel better about myself than I ever did before.

I was brought up in Hollywood, land of glamour and youth. At the age of twenty, I became involved in a singing career. Between singing jobs I worked in several Beverly Hills salons owned by a woman who taught me how to give facials and do makeup work, using her own customized cosmetic line. My two careers evolved side by side, and as a result of the learning process they took me through, I was motivated to write this book.

Because I had to learn to overcome my own fears plus the constant brainwashing of our youth-obsessed society, I had to prove to myself that I would not be "over the hill" by the time I was thirty or thirty-five. Since there was so much I wanted to do, and time was not standing still, I had to find a way to be ageless—physically, emotionally, and mentally. I sought out—and found—wonderful teachers from different parts of the world who taught me about facial massage, facial exercise, and skin care techniques. I also learned how to condition the rest of my body, as well as my mind, with the use of good nutrition, dance, tennis, yoga, and meditation, and the Pilates method. Joseph Pilates was the innovator of this state-of-the-art body conditioning system. He created a unique method of well-designed movements to increase the flexibility, strength, centering, and all-over longevity of the body. There are now more and more people involved in this wonderful body work.

After experimenting successfully on myself, I decided to take the best of my findings and teach what I had learned to other people and see if they achieved the same great results. Rather than giving facials one at a time, I decided to start teaching a class in order to show people how to give themselves facials every day. I kept perfecting and editing the technique so that it could become an automatic part of a person's daily routine. After all, what good is a technique if it is too drawn out or complicated for a person to use every day?

The results were fantastic. Everyone who used the technique started seeing a difference within the first few weeks.

At the same time, I had been developing a line of special natural skin care products to be used by my students. I didn't know at the time that these products would take off and develop an ardent following among users all over the world. I *did* begin to find that I was so busy getting my products out to the people that I had no time left to teach my classes. I finally decided that the only way to share my technique and make it more available to people would be in the form of a book.

In the meantime, my musical career also changed direction quite a bit. I discovered that I had a talent for songwriting. My songs started to be recorded by major artists; at the same time, I was teaching these celebrities valuable techniques for preserving a youthful appearance. This shows that there are no limitations on combining different forms of creativity, or on having more than one career.

My psychological attitudes about aging did not change overnight. However, my desire was to grow and to expand my awareness, because I was motivated to change the "neurotic destiny" I had thought was mine at a very early age. For this reason, I can tell you with certainty that you too can change your so-called destiny, revitalize your entire being—and reverse the aging process not only of your face, but of your mind and body as well.

Wishing you health, beauty,
and joy forever,

Rachel Perry

Reverse the Aging Process of Your Face

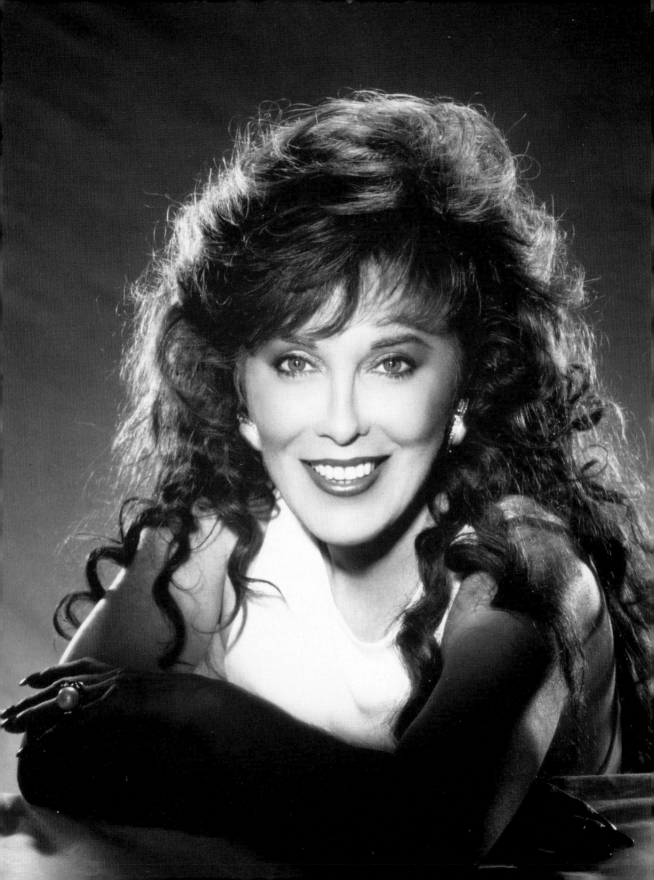

CHAPTER 1

A Simple Technique That Works

I am going to begin this book by restating the title—*Reverse the Aging Process of Your Face: A Simple Technique That Works*. It is the subtitle I now want to draw your attention to. Simplicity and effectiveness are the keys to the success of my technique. Because I am so involved in skin care, I read just about every new article and book on the subject. It almost always seems to me that the theories and techniques are long and drawn out, and many times too complicated for the average person to utilize. My bottom line is that there are a few very basic, but vitally important, steps to take that will help you achieve and preserve a young-looking, healthy skin, no matter what your age or skin type.

Most books on the subject of skin care leave out the vital points. Instead, they give a multitude of cosmetic recipes and superficial cleansing techniques that may give your skin a temporary "new" feeling, but that offer no lasting benefits. My purpose here is to give you a technique that will last a lifetime, and a book that you will not

"Each time you apply anything to your face, you can strengthen your facial muscles and rejuvenate your skin—easily and effectively. With your very own hands, you can reverse the aging process."

have to plow through to get the essential points.

In the course of my experience teaching facial rejuvenation to both women and men, and in the time I have spent developing my skin care line, I have found that there is a great deal of misinformation dealt out to the consumer concerning skin massage and the delicacy of skin tissue. This has resulted in what I call the "Overly Protective– No Benefit School of Skin Care." I have seen many people approach their faces with fear in their hearts—fear of stretching skin tissue, fear of irritating skin, and fear of pulling muscles. Because of this misinformation, many people's facial muscles and skin tissue lose their elasticity and remain out of condition, just like out-of-condition body muscles. If they can afford it, people with prematurely aging faces line up in the offices of plastic surgeons to have face-lifts as early as ten, twenty, and sometimes even thirty years before their time—and all because they didn't know a few simple preventive methods to include in their daily routines.

I now want to give you a brand-new point of view on the subject, and a brand-new skin to look forward to. My approach has resulted in great success for my students. It comprises a combination of facial exercise and what I call *epidermabrasion*, which is also known as exfoliation (sloughing or massaging the skin with friction), along with the application of scientifically designed skin care products. It does *not* consist of an endless series of complicated and time-consuming exercises that today's fast-paced lifestyles would not permit. Once you learn the few simple isometric facial positions and massage movements, you can use them whenever you apply anything to your face, from cleanser and scrub to moisturizer, night cream, and even make-up base. They can even be done while toweling dry. Herein lies the key to success with my technique. Each time you apply anything to your face, you will be strengthening your facial muscles and rejuvenating your skin. Think it sounds easy? It is.

THE HEALING AND REGENERATING POWER
IN OUR HANDS

The outer skin (the *epidermis*) is shedding all the time, roughly a layer of skin a day. The epidermis consists of about thirty layers in all. As the outer layers are being shed, new layers are also being formed at the base of the skin every day. As the skin ages, there is a normal slowing down of cellular reproduction. If the top shedding layers of skin are not promptly removed, the growth process and the formation of new skin tissue are slowed down even more. This leaves the complexion tired and muddy-looking. The skin loses its youthful vitality and, in short, ages faster. But don't give up hope! The good news is that by epidermabrading the skin tissue and removing those top shedding layers, you can actually speed up the process of cellular replacement and reproduction. In other words, with your very own hands, you will be reversing the aging process.

The power of human touch has been known for centuries by Asian, Native American, and many other cultures in which metaphysical thought is highly valued. There is a special heat that is generated from your own hands. This causes a deep electrical connection and opens up a flow of energy that reinforces every massage movement and increases all-over muscle toning. This is why there is a big difference between using electronic facial exercise machines and using your own hands. The life force energy your hands generate makes a real difference in achieving deeper and more long term results. It may seem a bit esoteric or abstract, but in all my experience of testing, experimenting, and using different methods (mainly due to my own insatiable curiosity), I have found that all mechanical and/or electrical tools seem to fall short of the simple use of my own hands, combined with the use of massage and isometric facial positions.

You can do a simple experiment by placing a small amount of any cosmetic cream in the palm of one hand and rubbing your hands together briskly for a minute. Feel the heat and energy your hands gen-

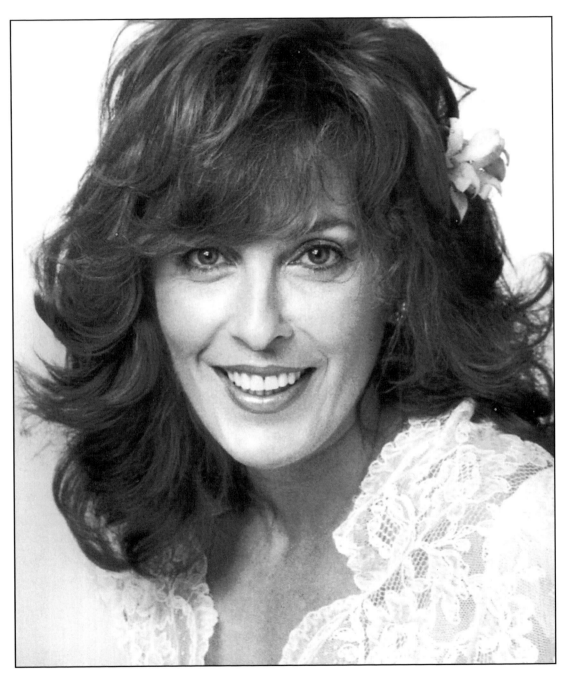

This is a picture of me in 1975 . . .

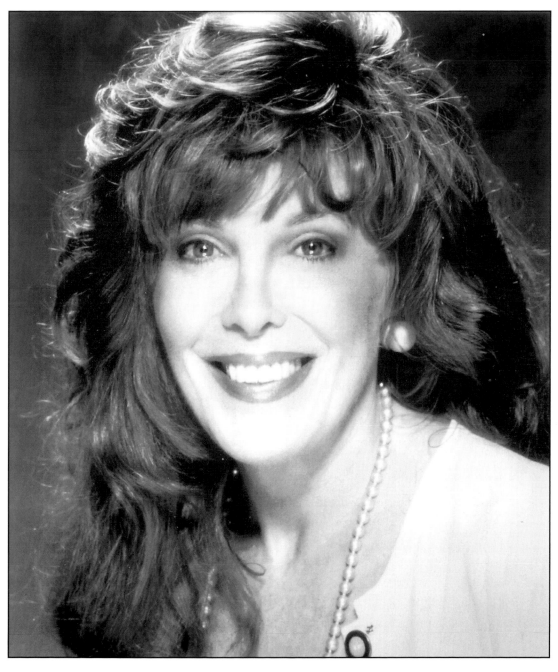

. . . and here I am today. Notice that the muscle definition in
the cheekbones is higher, the lips are fuller, and the jawline is
more well defined than in the photo taken twenty years ago.

erate. When you massage your face or body, you are transmitting this heat and life force energy to your own facial or body muscles. I am always open to new technology, but I also know that most of us are really unaware of the powerful ways in which our very own basic life force energy can bring about dramatic, ongoing, and long-lasting results.

By doing my massage you will automatically boost blood circulation to the area. You will also energize important acupressure points that stimulate the activity of the lymphatic system. The lymphatic system acts as the body's "sewer system"; it is the means by which wastes are carried away from the cells. Blood and lymphatic circulation work together to increase both the elimination of harmful toxins and the supply of oxygen and nutrients to the tissues. The ultimate result is improved and strengthened muscle tone.

EPIDERMABRASION

Consider the following interesting observation: Men rarely get the fine lines above the upper lip that are frequently present on mature women's faces. Why? I believe it is because most men shave every day, automatically epidermabrading that area and renewing the skin tissue. Many of the world's top dermatologists now agree that epidermabrasion (or exfoliation) is an absolute must for achieving translucent, smooth skin. Excellent results are being obtained not only with the problems of dry and aging skin, but also with overly oily skin that is prone to blackheads, and even with troubled, acne-prone skin. The mechanics of epidermabrasion aid in loosening oily plugs in the pores and unblocking them. This allows the pores to be emptied of secretions, and embedded toxic matter to be released more easily. Even if you have never heard the words *epidermabrasion*, *exfoliation*, or *sloughing* before, once you see the results on your own skin, I am sure you will never forget them.

My facial technique is simply this: You contract a facial muscle, hold it tense, and massage the area of the skin overlying it with friction. You will strengthen and improve both the skin and muscle tone this way. In the book *Face Culture*, Dr. Frederick Rossiter, a specialist in facial anatomy, says, "By contracting the muscle, the skin is not stretched or loosened and it is safe to massage away wrinkles and encourage circulation at the same time."[1]

Remember, good circulation is the most important factor in having a young-looking face. Improving circulation increases the supply of oxygen to the skin cells, which medical science agrees is one of the greatest and most important anti-aging factors. Along with boosting the amount of available oxygen, increased circulation results in more needed nutrients being carried to the skin and promotes the growth of healthy new skin cells. An increased blood supply close to the surface of the skin promotes the release of accumulated toxins that are lodged in the skin tissue, allowing the skin to "breathe" more freely.

More than once in my life, I have seen ballet dancers who are getting on in years who have the youngest looking bodies and the oldest looking faces. Why? Because they applied the basic principles of muscle toning and rejuvenation to every part of their bodies *except* their faces. It is this giant omission that I am endeavoring to correct with my technique. You can now look forward to the years ahead, knowing that you can have a young-looking face at any age. I think that is a very exciting prospect, don't you?

"Ever wonder why aging ballerinas often have young-looking bodies and old-looking faces? It's because they work on toning all the muscles in bodies—except for the ones in their faces. With a few simple exercises, you can look forward to having a young-looking face at any age."

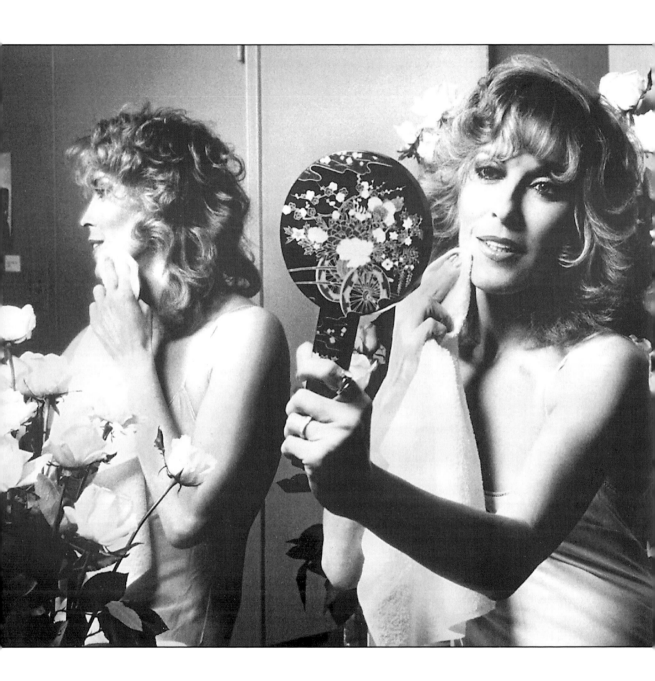

CHAPTER 2

Ready, Get Set . . . Glow!

My age-reversal process involves a sequence of four facial exercises combined with massage techniques. You should do the exercises as part of your daily skin care routine, using appropriate skin care products (for an outline of the basics of a good skin care routine, see Table 2.1 at the end of this chapter). Although you should use the exercise positions whenever you put anything on your skin (with the exception of masks and toners), there are two types of products that are really fundamental to the technique: cleansers and scrubs.

CLEANSERS

To do the first step of the program, the cleansing massage, you will use either a good creamy cleanser or a foaming facial cleansing gel or lotion that has a rich and full-bodied consistency. The most important property to look for when choosing a cleanser to use with my technique is its texture. It should have a spreadable enough consistency and enough body so that when it is applied to your face, your fingers move easily over your skin. This is necessary in order for the massage movements to reach deep into the muscles. To evaluate a cleansing product, place a small amount on your face and massage the area with your fingertips. If your fingers move easily, and the product remains on the skin surface instead of being absorbed into your skin, the cleanser has the right kind of consistency. If the cleanser soaks into your skin quickly, try another product that has more lubricity.

You will follow your cleansing massage by toweling off the cleansing cream, using the same positions and movements, or by rinsing off the foaming facial cleanser and then toweling dry, using the same positions and movements with the towel (more about towels later in this chapter).

SCRUBS

The second step, the scrub-massage, is a repeat of the first, except that this time, you will be using a good abrasive facial scrub in place of the cleanser or facial cleansing gel. Try to find a facial scrub made with as many natural ingredients as possible. These are most likely to be found in your local health food store. In my experience, the two primary ingredients that make for a great scrub are sea kelp and sea salt. They have the necessary abrasive action, are antibacterial, and give a smooth, refined texture to the skin.

If you cannot find a facial scrub that features these elements as its major ingredients, then I suggest that you buy a box of sea salt and some granulated sea kelp and mix some of each into the scrub you have purchased. Add a small amount, about one-quarter teaspoon each of sea salt and sea kelp per ounce of purchased product.

Other excellent natural ingredients for scrub-type products are peach or apricot kernel shell seeds, cornmeal, and papaya extract.

They all have great purifying, rejuvenating, and refining properties when used in scrubs.

A good scrub will draw impurities from the skin, remove dead, dry skin cells, and stimulate healthy circulation. There are different types of scrubs, some with a finer grade of abrasive and others that are rougher. No matter what type of scrub you use, you will get the most abrasive effect if you use it on dry skin. I have found that if you dampen your fingertips with water first, the additional moisture gives the scrub more spreadability. If your skin is not too sensitive, you can leave your face dry before you start the scrub massage, but you should still dampen your fingers. When doing epidermabrasion, always remember that you are the best judge of how abrasive to be with your own skin. If your skin is extremely sensitive, use the scrub on damp skin or dilute the scrub with a small amount of water at first. As your skin tissue becomes stronger, it will tolerate greater abrasiveness, and you can gradually increase the scrub-to-water ratio. If you find that a scrub is too harsh for your skin even with a bit of water added, you might want to look for a scrub product that is formulated specifically for sensitive skin. I repeat, let your skin tell you how it feels. It is the combination of epidermabrasion and muscle toning that makes this technique work.

THE IMPORTANCE OF pH BALANCE

Whatever products you choose, you should *always* use products that are pH-balanced, because they give the skin extra protection from deterioration and premature aging. The skin has a natural protective barrier called the *acid mantle*. The acid mantle is a kind of natural, invisible film on the surface of the skin that protects it from such harmful agents as bacteria and environmental pollutants. Any substance that is highly alkaline—including many skin care products that are not pH-balanced—tends to destroy the acid mantle, thus causing it to lose its ability to maintain your skin's delicate balance.

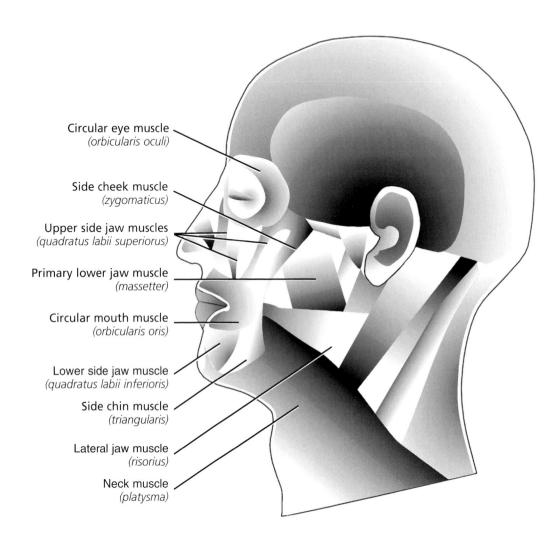

Circular eye muscle
(orbicularis oculi)

Side cheek muscle
(zygomaticus)

Upper side jaw muscles
(quadratus labii superiorus)

Primary lower jaw muscle
(massetter)

Circular mouth muscle
(orbicularis oris)

Lower side jaw muscle
(quadratus labii inferioris)

Side chin muscle
(triangularis)

Lateral jaw muscle
(risorius)

Neck muscle
(platysma)

Muscles Used in the Rachel Perry Facial Exercises

My exercises are designed to strengthen specific muscles of the face that are important for maintaining a youthful appearance. Some of these are the muscles around the eyes, the jaw muscles, the muscles around the mouth, and the side cheek, chin, and neck muscles.

In young, resilient skin, the protective acid mantle is very strong, and even after the use of alkaline products the skin bounces back to its normal, slightly acidic state in a very short time. But as skin ages, it takes longer and longer to return to its slightly acidic, healthy state. By protecting the acid mantle, products that are pH-balanced help to keep the skin in its healthiest state at all times.

A WORD ABOUT TOWELS

The proper toweling procedure is important to the success of my technique. I recommend that you get yourself a supply of small rough, white cotton terry-cloth towels—enough to last between laundry days. Hand towels are probably the most convenient size to use, because they are large enough to get the job done but small enough to be easy to handle. You can keep washing your towels over and over. I have enough to last me a week; every week I throw all the dirty ones in the laundry and start over again. Set these towels aside as your special facial towels.

AND NOW, THE EXERCISES

Now that you have assembled your cleanser, scrub, and towels, you are ready to begin doing the exercises. There are four basic exercises in the routine, each designed to strengthen specific muscle groups (see illustration, page 14). While you are learning your new routine, you may want to stand in front of a mirror to be sure you are doing the exercises correctly. Don't be alarmed—they will probably look rather strange at first. However, in a very short time you will know the exercises by the way they feel, rather than having to look every time you do them.

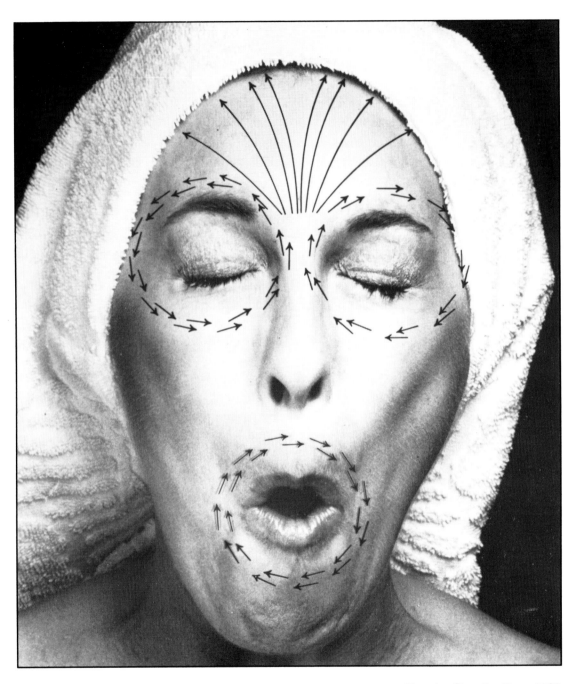

Exercise One: the Eternal "O"

Exercise One: The Eternal "O"

This exercise will keep the entire upper part of your face—including your nose, mouth, cheeks, and eye area—firm and uplifted. It will help prevent as well as slow down the gradual development of sagging skin and muscles. Your skin will become increasingly vital and glowing.

Exercise Position: Form a large oval "O" with your mouth, pulling your upper lip downward over your teeth. Now, without moving your mouth, smile, using the upper cheek muscles. At the same time, squeeze your eyelids tightly shut. (See illustration, page 16.) There should now be no loose skin tissue on your face, and you may massage your face energetically without worrying about pulling or stretching the skin.

Massage Technique: Holding the exercise position and using the fingertips of both hands, trace a complete circle around your eyes, starting always from the inner corners of your eyes and moving over your eyebrows, to the outer corners of your eyes, then under your eyes, including the upper cheeks, to complete a full circle. Do this a minimum of ten times, taking about one-half second to complete each circle. As your skin becomes more durable, you may want to increase the number of repetitions to as many as fifty to sixty.

Continue to maintain the exercise position and massage your nose with downward strokes about five times. Then, again using your fingertips, massage in a full circle around your mouth, making five full circles in one direction and then five full circles in the opposite direction.

Finally, place your fingertips at the bridge of your nose, and massage upward and outward over your forehead to your hairline, using five to ten long strokes.

The Eternal "O" will keep the upper part of your face firm and uplifted, preventing the development of sagging skin and muscles.

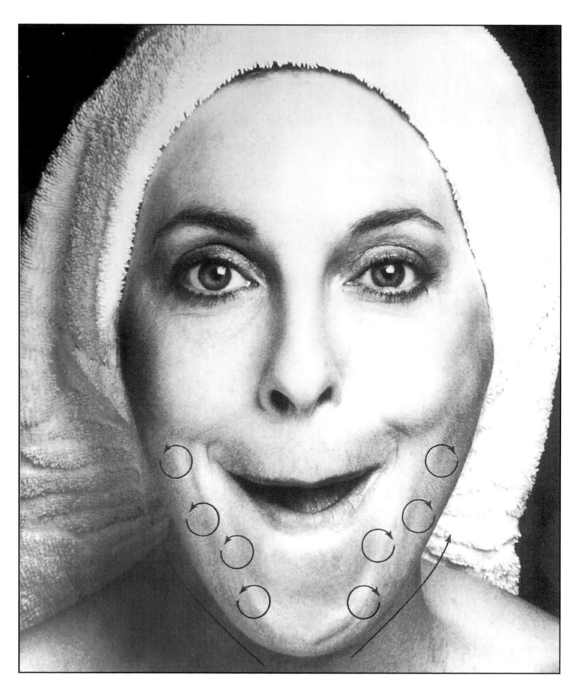

Exercise Two: the Firming Smile

Exercise Two: The Firming Smile

This exercise is for the bottom half of your face. It will keep the entire lower part of your face firm, preventing and correcting jowls and double chin problems.

Exercise Position: Roll your lips inward over your upper and lower teeth, leaving a space of about one-half inch between your lips. Now smile as widely as you can with your lower jaw. (See illustration, page 18.) It should feel as if your lower lip is smiling all the way to your ears. The rest of your face should remain unmoved.

Massage Technique: Holding the exercise position and using the fingertips of both hands, massage the entire lower part of your face in small outward circular motions. Starting at the tip of your chin, move up to your ears and then back down again, to a slow count of ten—or, if you are more ambitious, twenty.

The Firming Smile will keep the bottom half of your face firm and smooth, preventing the development of jowls and double chin.

Exercise Three: The Neck Rejuvenator

As its name implies, this third exercise will keep your neck muscles firm and your neck tissue smooth.

Exercise Position: Place your thumb under your chin and curl your tongue back in your mouth until you feel the muscle directly under your chin protrude. Now you may release your thumb, but continue to keep your tongue curled back in your mouth. Next, with your chin pointing upward, stretch your neck as far to the left as possible, to a

Exercise Three:
the Neck Rejuvenator

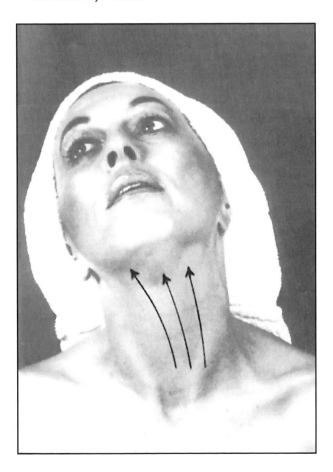
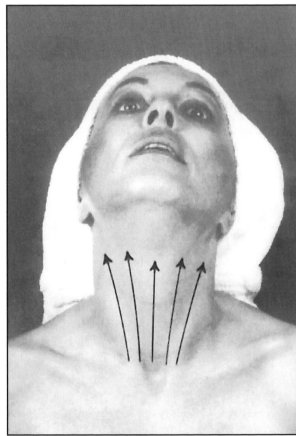

slow count of ten. Then slowly rotate to the opposite side. (See illustrations, below.)

Massage Technique: Placing the tips of the fingers of both hands at the base of your neck, massage in vigorous long, upward strokes from the base of your neck to your jawbone. Do this to a slow count of ten, while you are moving your neck in a half-circle arc from one side to the other.

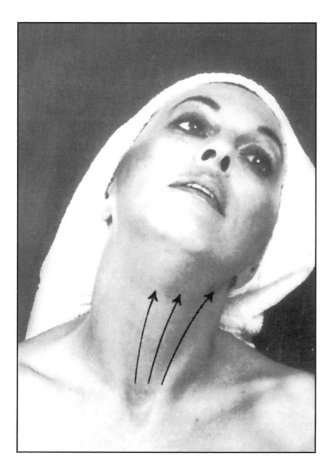

The Neck Rejuvenator will keep your neck firm, smooth, and youthful-looking.

Exercise Four, Step One:
The Upper Lip Smoother

This exercise will help
prevent those lines above
the lip from forming.

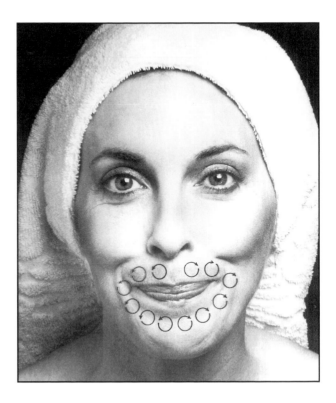

Exercise Four, Step Two:
The Around-the-Mouth
Strengthener

As its name implies,
this exercise will firm
the muscles around the
mouth. It will also firm
and fill out the lips.

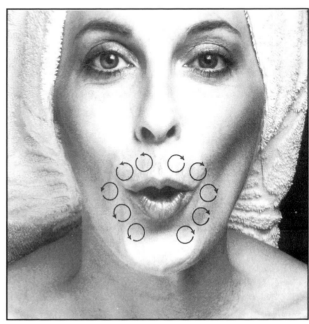

Exercise Four: The Upper Lip Smoother and Around-the-Mouth Strengthener

This exercise will do wonders for preventing and smoothing upper lip lines, smoothing those furrows that run from the corners of the mouth to the chin, strengthening the muscles around the mouth, and firming and filling out the lips.

Exercise Positions and Massage Technique: Press your lips together in a straight line, smiling slightly. Using the index fingers of both hands simultaneously, massage in tiny outward circular motions around the mouth. (See illustration, page 22, above.) Do this to a slow count of ten. Keep squeezing your lips together harder and harder, until you feel a tingling sensation around the mouth muscles.

Then immediately make a small "O" with your mouth, as if you were puckering up for a kiss, and smile very slightly. Continue to pucker harder and harder and massage in tiny outward circular motions around your mouth, counting again slowly to ten. (See illustration, page 22, below.) Then release.

Do this exercise at least twice a day with the massage, and whenever you can without the massage. You can even do it (without the massage) while you are driving, cooking, cleaning, reading, etc. It will soon become automatic, and it is well worth the effort.

Always remember to do the exercise positions and massage techniques every single time you apply cleanser and scrub. For the best results, you should also do them when you apply moisturizer, night cream, and even makeup base—anything that allows your fingers to move smoothly over your face. The exercises will soon become totally automatic and you won't even have to think about them. You *will* notice your skin being more receptive to moisturizers and nourishing creams and obtaining a gorgeous new glowing, youthful look.

Table 2.1 Step-By-Step Facial Care and Products

The facial exercises and massage techniques discussed in this chapter are meant to be used as part of your skin care routine. You should use them whenever you put anything on your skin (with the exception of masks and toners). The table below outlines the procedures and products for the eight steps of a good basic skin care routine, depending on your skin type.

SKIN TYPE	FIRST STEP	SECOND STEP	THIRD STEP	FOURTH STEP
	CLEANSING	EPIDERMABRADING & TIGHTENING	RETEXTURING & BALANCING	TONING
Normal and Combination Skin	Cleansing cream or foaming cleansing gel, followed by towel massage (every day).	Facial scrub (every day). Alternate between two different products, one more abrasive, the other less abrasive.	Clay-based mask (three times a week).	Skin toner without alcohol or astringent (every day). For combination skin, use astringent for oily T-zone, toner for drier cheek area.
Dry, Very Dry, and Aging Skin	Cleansing cream, followed by towel massage (every day).	Facial scrub (every day). Alternate between two different products, one more abrasive, the other less abrasive.	Clay-based mask (twice a week).	Skin toner without alcohol (every day).
Oily or Acne-Prone Skin	Foaming cleansing gel, followed by towel massage (every day).	Facial scrub (twice daily). Alternate between two different products, one more abrasive, the other less abrasive.	Clay-based mask (every day).	Alternate between antiseptic liquid skin toner and astringent (two or three times daily or when skin feels oily).
Sensitive Skin	Cleansing cream, followed by towel massage (every day).	Facial scrub (every other day). Choose a gentle formula designed for sensitive skin. If skin is extra sensitive, dilute the scrub with water.	Clay-based mask (once a week).	Skin toner without alcohol (every day).

If you are unsure about what type of skin you have, see Know Your Skin Type on page 34.

Keep in mind that this chart is meant to be a handy guide, not an inflexible set of rules. For example, if your normal skin is feeling dryer than usual one day, and you would like to apply an extra dose of moisturizer, go ahead. Similarly, just because a product may be called a night cream, that doesn't mean you can't use it during the day if you want to (just be sure to apply a sunscreen in addition to protect against the sun).

FIFTH STEP	SIXTH STEP	SEVENTH STEP	EIGHTH STEP
FIRMING	SPECIAL TREATMENTS	DAYTIME MOISTURIZING	NIGHTTIME NOURISHING
Skin-firming water-based gel primer (morning and evening).	Liposome eye/neck gel-cream; alpha-hydroxy acid skin serum, cream, or lotion; lip care product; and/or other special treatment, depending on individual needs (morning and evening).	Moisturizer (every morning). Alternate between two different products, one for normal skin, the other an oil-free moisturizer (see Chapter 4).	Nourishing treatment cream (every evening). For combination skin, use on dry areas and neck only. Alternate between two or more products with different nourishing ingredients (see Chapter 4).
Skin-firming water-based gel primer (morning and evening).	Liposome eye/neck gel-cream; alpha-hydroxy acid skin serum, cream, or lotion; lip care product; and/or other special treatment, depending on individual needs (morning and evening).	Moisturizer (every morning; reapply again during the day). Choose a maximum moisture formula with excellent hydrating ingredients (see Chapter 4).	Nourishing treatment cream (every evening). Alternate between two or more different products with different nourishing ingredients (see Chapter 4).
Skin-firming water-based gel primer (morning and evening).	Liposome eye/neck gel-cream; alpha-hydroxy acid skin serum, cream, or lotion; lip care product; and/or other special treatment, depending on individual needs (morning and evening).	Moisturizer (every morning). Choose an oil-free, noncomedogenic (non-pore-clogging) formula.	Massage nourishing treatment cream around eyes and on neck (every evening). Alternate between two or more different products with different nourishing ingredients (see Chapter 4).
Skin-firming water-based gel primer (morning and evening).	Liposome eye/neck gel-cream; alpha-hydroxy acid skin serum, cream, or lotion; lip care product; and/or other special treatment, depending on individual needs (morning and evening).	Moisturizer (every morning). Alternate between two different formulas, one maximum moisture, the other for normal skin.	Nourishing treatment cream (every evening). Alternate between two or more products with different nourishing ingredients (see Chapter 4).

The Role of Dentistry in Facial Rejuvenation

Dr. Peter Stone, a highly acclaimed dentist in California who specializes in cosmetic dentistry, recommended that I make my readers aware of the very important part that dental care plays in the goal of fighting facial aging. My facial exercise and massage technique is all about reversing aging by strengthening the facial muscles. However, no matter how diligent you are about caring for your skin and facial muscles, you cannot successfully reverse the aging process if you neglect to care for your teeth. The muscles of the face depend upon the teeth for their stability and support. When teeth are lost and not replaced by a partial denture, bridge, or dental implants, what occurs within the next few years of neglect is facial collapse.

In the dental arch, teeth depend on other teeth for stability. The muscles of the face also depend on that stability. To be more graphic, when there is no support for the facial muscles, wrinkles and depression lines form above and below the lips. The lips appear thin and flattened; the chin moves upward and outward and becomes more pointed; pouches form on either side of the lower jaw. Look at the drawings on page 27. They will probably remind you of faces you have seen before. A combination of good dentistry and my simple exercise techniques to strengthen the facial muscles can help prevent this from ever happening to you.

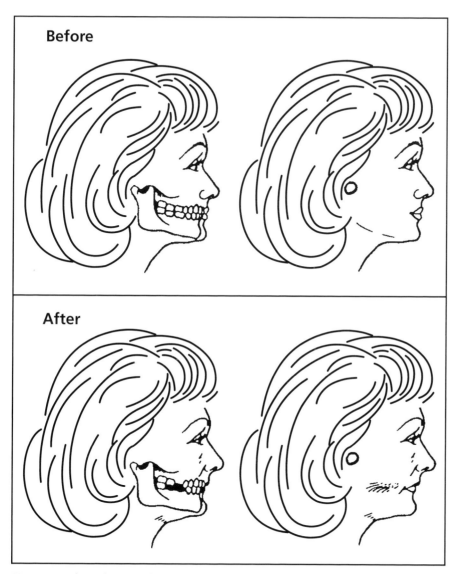

Before

After

How Dental Neglect Leads to Facial Aging

In the normal mouth, the teeth support the facial muscles (see the drawing above, left), making for a smooth facial contour (above, right). However, if teeth are lost and not replaced by partial dentures or dental implants (below, left), the muscles are not properly supported, and facial sagging and wrinkling result (below, right).

CHAPTER 3

Facial Cleansing—
The Whole Story

If, like most of us, you have read about and utilized other skin care regimens, you probably know that the first step is always a pre-scribed cleansing procedure. Lucky for you, you are now em-barking on a technique where the cleansing procedure not only cleans your skin, but also rejuvenates your skin tissue and the entire muscular structure of your face. In addition, because you are cleansing as part of this technique, your skin will become normalized and better balanced. If your skin is on the dry side, the increased cir-culation will stimulate the oil glands to work more efficiently; if it is on the oily side, clogged pores will be unblocked and the excess oil drained and controlled, rather than wreaking havoc with your face.

THE CLEANSING MASSAGE

As described in Chapter 2, the first step in my skin care technique involves using a good pH-balanced cleansing cream or a foaming facial cleansing gel or lotion to give yourself a cleansing massage.

The cleansing massage combines a deep cleansing with the benefits of exercise and massage, strengthening the muscle tone and stimulating circulation. There are several good creamy cleansers on the market that are water soluble, which means that they can be used with water as a face wash if you have oily skin (or if you simply prefer washing your face for an initial cleansing). Whatever cleanser you use, the second step—the scrub-massage—will give you a good rinsing-off anyway. Do the cleansing massage, following the exercise and massage instructions in Chapter 2.

If you wear makeup, you should first use the cleanser to remove makeup and then reapply the cleanser to start the cleansing massage. In other words, if you wear makeup, the first application and removal of cleanser are done *before* starting the actual technique.

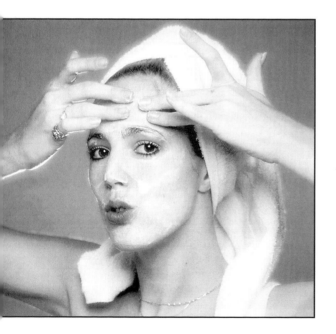

Begin the cleansing massage with the Eternal "O."

You wouldn't want to massage old makeup into your skin, would you? The same principle applies if your skin feels grimy or dirty; give it a quick once-over first with the cleanser and rinse it off. Then reapply the cleanser and start the cleansing massage. This will allow you to maintain excellent skin hygiene.

I have not used bar soap to cleanse my face in many years. Most bar or cake soaps have always been highly alkaline and capable of stripping the skin of its protective acid mantle. I personally never liked the feeling that bar soaps left on my skin, so I never use them. However, certain formulators of bar soaps have made some wonderful improvements in their technology, so even though I am still not a bar soap user myself, I cannot honestly say that every single one of them is a no-no. Some of the newer bar soaps can be quite good. It is always good to stay open to evolving biochemistry.

What I do use, however—and love to alternate with my cleansing cream as a cleanser—is a good pH-balanced foaming facial cleansing gel or lotion. If you like to wash your face and get a sudsing effect, a foaming cleansing gel or lotion that is pH-balanced and contains good natural ingredients may be the answer for you. Not only is it okay to use one, but I have found—much to my delight—that if the consistency of the foaming facial cleanser has a good amount of richness and body, it can be used instead of, or alternated with, a facial cleansing cream for the massage.

TOWELING

The toweling procedure is very important to understand. At the end of your cleansing massage, repeat the exercise positions as you towel off, using one of your rough white terry-cloth towels (if you are using a rinse-off facial cleansing product, leave your face wet and then towel dry). Start with one end of a clean white towel and follow the massage techniques, using the towel this time instead of your fingers. After finishing with the first part of your face, move to a clean part of the towel and do the next part of your face. For example, if your face is in the Eternal "O" position, you would start with your right eye and make a full circle around the eye with the towel. Then you would move to a clean piece of towel and proceed to the left eye. As you move through each area of your face—your

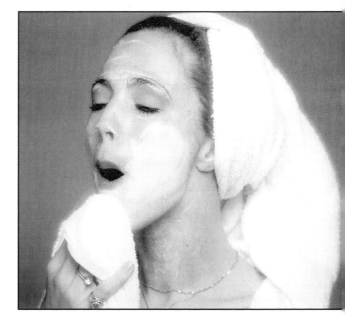

Repeat the exercise positions and massage movements with the towel.

nose, around your mouth, your forehead, etc.—keep moving the towel to a clean spot. One towel can go a long way (remember, you can use both sides). By doing this you will not only get a good circulation boost from the towel massage, but you will also know exactly how much dirt and grime was left on your face. When that white towel stays white, you will know your skin is clean, and you can go on to the second step, the scrub-massage. If, however, there is still grime showing on the towel, reapply your cleanser and once again towel off or rinse and towel dry.

THE SCRUB-MASSAGE

Apply your facial scrub with dampened fingertips.

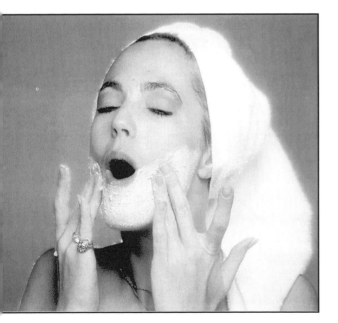

The second step of my technique, the scrub-massage, is what gives your pores a deep, thorough cleansing. I never feel that my cleansing is complete until after I do my scrub-massage. This is the step in which the deep, stubborn impurities are drawn out and the dead, dry layers of skin are removed, leaving the skin like satin.

Using your facial scrub, repeat the exercise positions and massage techniques once again. I suggest dampening your fingertips to give the scrub the most spreadability and to allow for easier movement of your fingers when doing the scrub-massage. You are now ready to rinse. Rinse with warm to very warm water—in fact, as warm as your skin can take comfortably (no burns, please). Rinse several times until your skin is totally clean. Warm water is wonderful for increasing the flow of blood in the tissues and stimulating the oil glands in the skin to work more efficiently. This is good for both oily and dry skin problems; it loosens deep-seated toxins in the pores (for oily skin), and generally enlivens skin tone (for dry skin).

TONING

You may now apply a toning product to your skin. There are three basic types: toners, astringents, and antiseptics. Toners are liquids that remove any remaining traces of dirt and grime, giving your skin a clarified and fresh appearance. Astringents do all of that, but also have oil-controlling properties. Often, they contain a small amount of alcohol. The antiseptic types of toner or astringent also kill bacteria. They almost always contain some amount of alcohol. If you have a

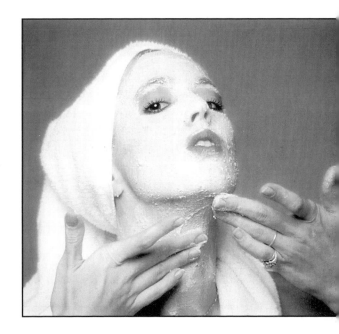

Step three of the scrub-massage: the Neck Rejuvenator.

normal or combination skin type (see page 34), you may use either toner or astringent. If you have dry skin, you should use a skin toner; if you have oily skin, an astringent is appropriate. If your skin is acne-prone, you should use an antiseptic type of astringent.

Toning encourages the pores to tighten up again after the "grand opening" pore cleansing of the scrub-massage. Whatever type of toning product you use, be sure to find one that is pH-balanced. This is very important for restoring your skin to its proper and protected acid balance (see page 13). Toners may be swept over the skin on a cotton ball, or splashed on, as after-shave. Some come in spray bottles. Follow the application directions on the product you choose. I have found that keeping toner or astringent in the refrigerator during warm or hot weather adds a wonderfully

Know Your Skin Type

In order to choose skin care products, it is helpful to have some idea of your basic skin type. Skin is usually classified as normal, dry, or oily. Other skin types that are sometimes mentioned are combination skin (skin that has both dry and oily areas), sensitive skin, and mature skin. The table below can help you evaluate what your skin is like and which products may be best for you. Please keep in mind, however, that this is meant to be a guide, not a straitjacket. Skin types overlap a great deal, and everyone's skin changes over time. As you work with the exercise and massage techniques and experiment with different products, use your own judgment to decide what your skin is like and which products perform best for you.

SKIN TYPE	CHARACTERISTICS
Normal Skin	No excessive oiliness, even in T-zone (forehead, nose, and chin areas) Retains moisture—no dry or "tight" feeling Smooth texture
Dry, Very Dry, and Aging Skin	Thin skin, fine pores Dryness, flakiness Fine lines Roughness Tight, uncomfortable feeling Dull appearance
Oily or Acne-Prone Skin	Enlarged pores Shiny appearance within an hour after cleansing Tendency to feel greasy to the touch Breakouts and blackheads

SKIN TYPE	CHARACTERISTICS
Combination Skin	Oily skin in T-zone (forehead, nose, and chin areas) Dry or normal skin in cheek and eye area
Sensitive Skin	Irritation Redness or blotchiness Itchiness Extra sensitivity to the sun

refreshing bonus to the benefits you can receive from these products.

After doing the basic daily cleansing procedure—the cleansing massage, the scrub-massage, and toning—for a few weeks, you will find that the fresh new vitality of your skin will motivate you to make a habit of it.

CHAPTER 4

Moisturizing and Nourishing a Thirsty, Hungry Skin

It may seem a bit strange to think of your skin as being thirsty or hungry, but it is an accepted fact among biochemists and dermatologists that all skin needs both moisture *and* nutrients. Even if your skin is oily, it may still lack moisture. When skin is overly oily, it is because the sebaceous glands are too active. This has nothing to do with the skin's ability to retain moisture, which refers to the water present in the skin tissue.

MOISTURIZERS: A DRINK FOR THIRSTY SKIN

The outer layers of the skin are called the *stratum corneum*. The stratum corneum is ten to twenty layers deep. It is fed from within the body, but it does not retain much water, especially as the skin ages. The younger the skin, the more moisture this outer layer retains.

Moisturizers are necessary because they act on these outer layers. A good moisturizing cream or lotion will both prevent excessive evaporation of moisture from the surface of the skin and also add water to it. Moisturizers contain agents called humectants that increase the skin's ability to hold water in. One of the best humectants is hyaluronic acid (sodium hyaluronate), which has a tremendous water-holding capability. This substance occurs naturally in our own skin, but the amount that is present decreases as we age. Skin care chemists and dermatologists call hyaluronic acid the "super-hydrator" because it has the incredible ability to attract, hold, and bind 1,000 times its own weight in water. In adequate quantities, researchers say, it can bind more water to the skin than any other type of water-soluble moisturizing agent yet discovered. And when skin has this kind of ample moisture level, it has a plump, cushiony feel—like a baby's skin—and the texture is soft and supple. In the past, the only hyaluronic acid available for purchase was derived from the combs of roosters, but in an effort to get away from animal sources, this ingredient is now scientifically engineered by a microbiological process from a long chain of molecules derived from glucose. Hyaluronic acid from this new source is known to perform even better than the animal product. There has been no expense spared to create hyaluronic acid, since it has been found to be one of the most beneficial moisturizing ingredients in the world.

There are other moisturizing ingredients that work well in skin care formulas, too, such as red sea algae, sodium PCA (a protein derivative also known as NaPCA), tissue respiratory factor (TRF, which is also known as skin respiratory factor or SRF, and is derived from live yeast cells), and a number of different botanical extracts, including aloe vera, ginseng, calendula, suma, echinacea, and many more, all of which increase the skin's moisture level and help to retard moisture loss.

Since moisturizing cream is designed to lock in as well as to add moisture, it works best when applied on a damp or just-washed face, and is especially effective when used after applying a water-based facial gel (more about this later in this chapter). This way you utilize the product to its fullest extent, locking in a fresh supply of water while at the same time giving the skin a more supple and firm look and feel.

Another way to increase the moisture in your skin is to humidify the air in your bedroom. This can be done very easily by using a steam humidifier, a vaporizer, or even a pan of water placed on top of a radiator. This will help keep the air moist for hours and will benefit your respiratory system as well as your skin. Since many of us spend winters in heated rooms and summers in air-condition-ed rooms—both of which are severely drying climates—the humidifier is a real godsend. It gives you a moisturizing treat-ment while you sleep.

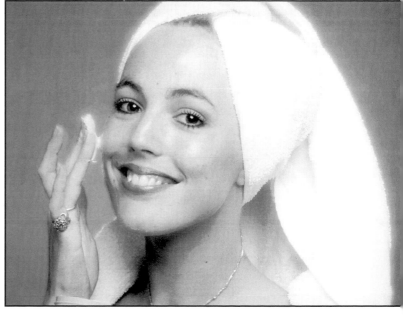

I live in California, where the air is always dry. I have met actresses from England who said that when they moved here, their once-beautiful skin started to wrinkle and dry out almost immediately, but they found that nighttime humidify-ing, along with the use of good creams, gave them back their beau-tiful English complexions. I especially recommend this technique to all people who spend a great deal of time in what could be the driest climate of all, the pressurized cabin of an aircraft. The air inside an airplane measures less than 3 percent humidity, making dry skin a constant problem. Whenever I fly, I make intermittent trips to the lavatory to dampen my face with a wet paper towel, apply my water-based gel, and then reapply my moisturizing cream. If you are an air-line flight attendant, or if you just do a lot of flying, this can be a great

Every skin, even oily skin, needs the benefits of a good moisturizer.

help. After all, it's no fun arriving at your destination feeling like your face has been out in the Gobi desert during a windstorm.

NOURISHING TREATMENTS: FOOD FOR HUNGRY SKIN

What, you may ask, is the difference between a moisturizing cream and a nourishing cream? The difference is in the way they are formulated. All creams and lotions are basically a combination of water and oil blended together in an emulsion. Moisturizers and gels are more concentrated with water; nourishing creams usually contain a higher concentration of oil. In addition to replenishing lost oil, they nourish the skin with elements that aid in encouraging the growth of healthy new skin cells. As we get older, our skin benefits more and more from these nourishing treatments. The basic oil keeps the outer skin supple and soft. Continual lubrication is an absolute must for young-looking skin! I especially like nourishing creams that contain ingredients to nourish skin that may have been deprived of proper lubrication, as well as ingredients to prevent such deprivation from happening in the first place.

Much research has been done on which elements do the best job, and there are now a number of great gels, creams, and serums on the market. Skin care science is always isolating new biological substances and finding new ways to use them for more effective moisturizing, nourishment, and overall improvement to help achieve the appearance of firmer, younger skin. There are some ingredients that contain soluble protein, created from chains of amino acids. Because these substances are soluble (mixable), they can be used very effectively in all treatment products. You may already be familiar with one of these substances, water-soluble collagen protein, which has been used by cosmetic manufacturers for a number of years. Water-soluble collagen protein represents one group of amino acids; science has also broken down its partner, hydro-elastin, which represents another group of amino acids. Both of these two groups of amino acids are water-soluble, and both are essential components of the dermis, the supportive skin tissue underlying the epidermis. They are responsible for the youthful resilience of the skin fibers. These valuable amino acid chains are plentiful in young skin, but start to diminish somewhere in a person's middle to late twenties. The result of this is a loss of the skin's elasticity.

With the discovery and isolation of hydro-elastin, we now have the opportunity to use both groups of amino acids. Natural skin science has now also been able to develop vegetable equivalents of both collagen and elastin, which were formerly available only from animal sources. In some of the best types of nighttime nourishing products, another substance, called mucopolysaccharide, is combined with hydro-elastin and water-soluble collagen protein to create a synergistic effect. Mucopolysaccharides can enhance the function of the elastin and collagen in the skin tissue, making them more effective in their ability to hold moisture in the outer layers of the skin.

"The great thing about liposomes is that they can deliver beneficial nutrients and other natural ingredients more effectively into all the layers of the skin."

LIPOSOMES

Skin care science now has ways of bringing needed nourishment deeper into the skin cells than ever before. These technologies and all that they encompass are called *delivery systems*. Delivery systems can make topical applications of moisturizers and nutrients as much as ten times more effective in their ability to penetrate deeply into the layers of the skin.

Perhaps the best and most often used delivery system in skin care today is liposomes. These liposomes are tiny particles capable of encapsulation. Their minute size permits almost immediate penetration of, and delivery of nutrients into (and beneath), the outer layers of the skin, the stratum corneum. (see illustration, page 42)

Liposomes are microscopic oblong spheres with a liquid center, like a tiny bubble. They can be used to encapsulate water and/or other substances that are beneficial for the skin. Since a liposome

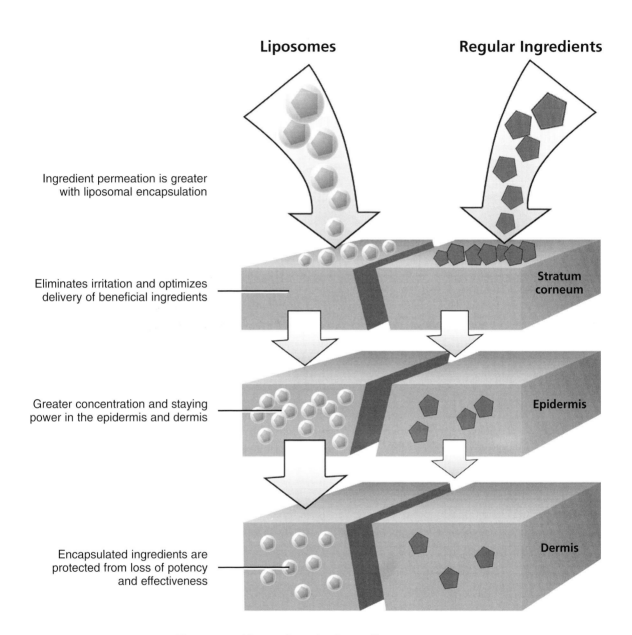

Liposomes

Regular Ingredients

Ingredient permeation is greater with liposomal encapsulation

Eliminates irritation and optimizes delivery of beneficial ingredients

Greater concentration and staying power in the epidermis and dermis

Encapsulated ingredients are protected from loss of potency and effectiveness

Stratum corneum

Epidermis

Dermis

Liposomes Versus Regular Ingredients

This illustration shows how liposomes can deliver ingredients deeper into the layers of the skin.

sphere is smaller than a skin cell, the core ingredient or ingredients in the center can be delivered and released into the skin precisely where needed and as needed. Liposomes are similar in structure to the membranes of our own skin cells, and because of this they can deliver to the skin superior moisturizing, lubricating, and nourishing ingredients such as humectants, vitamins, minerals, enzymes, trace elements, alpha-hydroxy acids, sunscreens, and even antioxidants. All these substances help to improve skin function as well as to fight the deterioration of skin cells brought about by the action of free radicals. Currently, the most often used ingredients include tissue respiratory factor (TRF), beta-glucan, superoxide dismutase (SOD), various vitamins, alpha-hydroxy acids, and now even new fat-reducing agents called methylxanthines. All of these are used to protect, repair, and regenerate damaged skin cells.

The outer shells of liposomes are composed of a type of lipid. These special lipids are oily substances called phospholipids or sphingolipids. The best are made from a natural oil, such as lecithin derived from soybeans or egg yolks. These phospholipids form a bilayer shell surrounding an internal compartment filled with an active ingredient, or several ingredients. Together, the outer shell and the internal compartment make up the liposome. Liposomes penetrate the surface of the skin, and once they do, the encapsulated ingredients are released, and the active ingredients, plus the lipid shell, are incorporated into all layers of the skin, including the stratum corneum, the living epidermis, and the dermis. The inner ingredients surrounded by the outer phospholipids are usually specifically chosen for their superior moisturizing and nourishing capabilities. Depending on the particular liposome structure, these ingredients can provide the skin with benefits for eight to twelve hours.

Liposomes can be incorporated into cleansers, creams, lotions, gels, gel-creams, serums, ointments, shampoos, and even makeup. This makes them very desirable for use in many, many skin care, cosmetic, and even hair care products. Just about every cosmetic company in the world (including my own) now uses liposomes in its formulations for moisturizers and night treatment creams, because liposomes have the ability to deliver active ingredients into deeper layers of the skin. There are even some timed-release liposome formulas that can release ingredients for as long as a twenty-four-hour period. This gives more impact to the beneficial hydrating and nourishing action of special skin care ingredients.

Dr. Brian C. Keller, director of research and development at BioZone Laboratories, Inc., says, "The topical application of "active" ingredients has become a major focus of users of skin care and cosmetic products. However, these actives must permeate into deeper layers of the skin to achieve their potential and maximize their benefits. The use of liposomes signals a revolutionary method of reformulating cosmetic products to improve efficacy, safety, and user acceptability."[1]

The use of liposomes in skin care products has been shown to aid in reducing and minimizing wrinkles and fine lines. Depending upon what ingredients the liposomes in any particular product contain, the benefits will vary. The great thing about this technology is that all the wonderful natural ingredients that I have always found to be beneficial, and all the new ingredients that skin care science has to offer, can now be integrated into liposome delivery systems.

SPECIAL NOURISHING TREATMENTS

Before we leave the subject of nourishing treatments, I would like to discuss two special types of products that are especially valuable for keeping skin well nourished: water-based gel formulas and special eye treatments. Both of these should be used in conjunction with regular moisturizers and nourishing creams for maximum benefit to your skin.

Water-Based Gel Formulas

Many people are amazed to learn that there are so many epidermal layers. In fact, there are somewhere between twenty-one and twenty-seven layers in all. Research has shown that the best carrier of some substances to the skin is simply water. Whereas certain oil-soluble substances are carried more effectively in an oil-based formula, other substances seem to have more of an effect on the skin when incorporated into a water-based gel formula. I like using water-based gel formulas for some products and oil-based cream formulas for other products. For instance, water-based gel products containing water-soluble collagen, hydro-elastin, and water-soluble infusions of botanicals are very effective.

"Think of water-based gel as a primer to precede the use of moisturizing and nourishing treatments."

The use of a water-based facial gel should be a part of your regime because water is easily absorbed into the dermis, giving an immediate fresh, firm, and supple feel and look to the skin. I think of water-based gel as a primer to precede the use of cream or lotion moisturizers and nourishing treatment products. Water-based gels are great for all skin types: dry, normal, or oily.

For best results, a water-based facial gel should be applied after cleansing and toning and before applying moisturizer or nourishing cream. After you apply a water-based facial gel and it is absorbed, follow it with an application of a special eye treatment (see page 46) and then your daytime moisturizer or nourishing night cream, or some other special treatment cream or serum. Using a water-based gel this way gives additional lubrication and nourishment to the skin while providing the emollient barrier necessary to lock in the water-soluble collagen, hydro-elastin, and water-soluble botanical extracts the gel contains.

Eye Treatments

The eye area is a special issue in skin care. It presents two distinctive problems. One is the delicacy of the skin tissue, which is thinner and therefore tends to crinkle and wrinkle sooner than the rest of the face. This thinner skin also has more difficulty retaining moisture and natural oils. The second problem with the eye area is its tendency to swell at the drop of a tear. You have probably noticed extra swelling around your eyes on many occasions—whether from "that time of the month," watching a good tear-jerker, a late evening with less than normal sleep, allergies, a sinus problem, exposure to smog or other irritants, water retention, or intestinal problems. I'm sure you get the picture.

I have always found the use of a good clay- or mud-based mask to be very effective in reducing under-eye swelling. (More about this in Chapter 5.) I have also found that the use of a gel or gel-cream can be very effective if it contains certain ingredients. Look for a formula that contains special botanicals such as calendula, chamomile, echinacea, marigold, sea algae, and sage. Other ingredients to look for include tissue respiratory factor (TRF), beta-glucan, elastin, collagen, mucopolysaccharides, and hyaluronic acid. These ingredients have nourishing, moisturizing, and anti-swelling properties, and can be very effective for this area that needs special attention. I like using an eye gel or gel-cream with these special botanicals in the morning, because that is when the most swelling seems to occur, and a gel gives the speediest and most visible improvement. It reduces the swelling and puffiness, thereby giving a tighter, firmer look to the skin around the eyes. I have also experienced good results by taking a washcloth, wetting it with very warm water (but not hot enough to scald the skin!), holding it right underneath my eyes, and pressing for a minute or two. Then I switch to an ice-cold wet washcloth, folded around an ice cube, and press that on the skin underneath my eyes for another couple of minutes. Alternating these treatments for about ten minutes in many cases helps to take swelling down. At night, I suggest using a high-powered eye treatment formula containing some of the great natural skin nutrients mentioned above to nourish this hungry and thirsty skin tissue. You should use your night cream or moisturizer on top of your eye cream, gel, or gel-cream, both day and night.

CHOOSING MOISTURIZERS AND NOURISHING CREAMS

When choosing products to moisturize and nourish your skin, it is important to select formulas made from the best possible ingredients. For example, if a product is a combination of oil and water, or has an oil base, it is a good idea to look at the type of oil it contains. The types of oils I think of as the best, and the ones that I've always preferred to use in my product formulas, are the natural vegetable oils, such as jojoba, sweet almond, safflower, avocado, sunflower, wheat germ, apricot kernel, sesame, evening primrose, borage, and canola. They are all rich in essential fatty acids (EFAs, also sometimes called unsaturated fatty acids), such as gamma-linolenic acid (GLA). EFAs are sometimes also referred to as "vitamin F." All of these oils are superior for enriching and smoothing the skin. Many commercial products use mineral oil or petrolatum as a base oil, but these substances can be highly occlusive (pore-clogging), and they have no nutritional value. The alternative is to use natural vegetable oils. These not only do the job of lubricating, but are treasure troves of vitamins and minerals as well. In addition to the oils mentioned above, there are also oils derived from the rain forests. They not only provide benefits for the skin, but the use of these oils in moisturizing and nourishing products creates new opportunities for the native peoples of rain forest regions to generate income without endangering their forests. Some of these oils now being used are kukui nut, Brazil nut, copaiba, orchid, babassu (palm kernel), and sapayul; many others are still being discovered.

"Caring for combination skin doesn't have to be confusing. Just treat the dry areas like dry skin, and the oily areas like oily skin."

Many vitamins—including A, C, D, and E, as well as the B vitamins—have been shown over and over to be a source of skin benefits. Royal bee jelly is an enriching substance that contains vitamins, minerals, and protein; bee pollen contains many vitamins, minerals, enzymes, DNA, and RNA. Squalane is a smoothing ingredient that has a remarkable satinizing effect on even the driest of skin. This ingredient used to be derived from shark liver, but now—fortunately for those of us who are against the use of animal byproducts—the same substance is being extracted from olives, and is just as effective, if not more so.

Shea butter, a rich and buttery substance from the African karite nut tree, and lecithin, an excellent skin enricher derived from soybeans, are also among the best natural skin-smoothing and nourishing ingredients. Other good ingredients include enzymes such as papain (from papaya) and bromelain (from pineapple), and earth minerals such as clay and mud. And last—but not least—are the botanicals (herbs and plant extracts) that stimulate and nourish the skin tissue. These include ginseng, ginkgo biloba, suma, aloe vera, agave, babassu (also known as palm kernel oil), copaiba, sapayul, echinacea, chamomile, sea algae, spirulina, and many different sea plant extracts. Consult Appendix I at the end of this book to find out more about nature's wonderful skin care ingredients and what they are known for.

You can't go wrong using creams, gels, masks, scrubs, and other skin care products that contain these natural substances to condition your skin. Experiment with different products to see which combination of ingredients seems to do the most for you and which textures feel the best. If your skin is very dry, you might prefer a very rich cream, or you might alternate this with a lighter textured cream every other night or day. If your skin is on the oily side, a good lightweight moisturizer may be enough, along with a richer cream or one specifically designed for the eye or neck area, both of which tend to become dry sooner than the rest of the face. There are many good oil-free moisture creams and lotions available now that give oily skin the benefit of moisture without excess oil.

Many people have combination skin—skin that is oily in some areas and dry in others. This is an issue that many people find confusing, and, in fact, I find that it comes up every time I lecture. Even though many cosmetic companies make it seem complicated, it is really quite simple: If you have combination skin, just treat the oily areas as you would oily skin, and treat the drier areas as you would dry skin. For example, if you have an oily "T-zone" (the area encompassing your forehead, nose, and possibly your chin) but you also have a problem with dryness around your eye area, you should simply cleanse, tone, and moisturize the T-zone with products designed for oily skin, and use products designed for dry skin on the skin around your eyes. It really is just that simple.

Another question that comes up frequently concerns the difference between day creams and night creams. Mostly, cosmetic companies designate moisturizing creams as being for daytime use and nourishing creams as being for nighttime use. The reasoning behind this is that moisturizers are known to counteract the drying elements in the air during the daytime. Also, more and more of these products now contain sunscreens to protect skin against damage from the sun's ultraviolet rays and from environmental pollutants, and they are usually light textured enough to wear under a makeup base or foundation. However, I personally do not feel a need to make this distinction between products on the basis of night and day, and see no reason not to use a nourishing night cream all day or a moisturizer at night, if that is what your skin needs (and you can always put a sun block on underneath any cream during the day). The skin needs both types of creams for complete care. Unless a night cream is too heavy or oily-looking to wear under makeup or out in public, go ahead and use it if you want to.

ALTERNATE YOUR TREATMENT PRODUCTS

This brings me to the subject of another question people ask frequently: "With all these wonderful products, which ones do I use and when do I use them?" I am a big exponent of *alternation of skin care treatment products*. I feel that one of the keys to having great-looking skin is alternating among a number of different products, so that the skin has all of its needs fulfilled. For example, if I use a moisturizer during the day, then I use a nourishing cream at night, and vice versa. This means continually alternating between moisturizing- and nourishing-type products. You may want to use one nourishing cream during the day and another one, with different ingredients, at night. Basically, you should just keep alternating among several different creams, gels, or special treatments that all offer different elements. Do the same thing with cleansing treatment products such as scrubs and cleansing creams.

It's just like varying your diet. You wouldn't eat the same exact meal three times a day, every day, would you? You need to get different nutrients from different foods. Just as your body would become bored and dulled if you ate the same menu day after day, your skin will become bored, dulled, deficient, and lackluster if you use exactly the same products day in and day out. Whichever part of your face you are dealing with, the philosophy is very simple. Each formula has its own particular attributes, and you want your skin to obtain all the benefits that science and nature have to offer. Variety is not only the spice of life—it is a vital and necessary part of achieving the kind of great skin you want to have.

Medical science has determined that our bodies need many different and vitally important vitamins, minerals, trace elements, proteins, enzymes, essential fatty acids (EFAs), and antioxidants in order to avoid deficiencies and keep our immune systems strong and healthy. We require a combination of many different nutritional substances to fulfill our bodies' requirements. A strong immune system makes for

"You wouldn't eat the same meal three times a day, every day, so why feed your skin that way?"

a healthy body. The skin—which is the body's largest organ—has the same requirements, but needs to be fed from the outside as well as from the inside.

There is also the matter of balance. For example, if you are doing a great amount of epidermabrasion, a good cream containing vitamin E can very quickly soothe, replenish, and smooth out any roughness that occurs after this skin workout. Every really good product has its own reason for being, and the greater the variety of ingredients you can use, the more your skin will benefit. Even if a product is not especially designed for my particular skin type, I may still use it from time to time if it contains certain ingredients that I know will be beneficial to my skin. I will alternate these other products with the products designed specifically for my skin type in order to receive the additional nutrients they offer. So, for example, even if you have oily skin and would not normally choose to use a super-rich cream, if you find a rich cream with great ingredients, you should use it on any areas where you see that fine, dry lines are starting to develop.

I am emphatic about product alternation because I have found that it yields immediate results that you can see for yourself. And remember, whichever gels, creams, lotions, gel-creams, serums, or any other products you use, and whatever skin type you have, always do the basic exercise positions and use the facial massage techniques when applying them. Nothing can take the place of doing the facial technique. This is what makes the big difference between partial skin care and really reversing the aging process.

CHAPTER 5

Peeling Away the Years—
Nature, Science, and Substances

For years I have been teaching and preaching about epidermabrasion (exfoliation) and its function in the rejuvenation and regeneration of the skin. The majority of dermatologists and skin care scientists now agree that the action of removing dead, dry skin cells from the surface layers actually does speed up the regeneration process of new cells rising to the surface. This action has been proven to help eliminate fine lines and premature wrinkling. As a result, skin care professionals are now recommending the use of a wide variety of agents to help the peeling process along.

RETIN-A

There are a number of substances that have been scientifically developed that have an effect on the skin similar to that of epidermabrasion. One of the best known of these is Retin-A.

Retin-A is a prescription product also known as retinoic acid or vitamin-A acid. The active ingredient is called tretinoin. This substance is a member of the family of vitamin-A compounds called retinoids. Retin-A was originally devised to lessen the scarring and eliminate the blockage of infected pores, blackheads, and whiteheads in patients with acne. It was later discovered that Retin-A also has the ability to dramatically improve the appearance of aging skin. It causes a peeling of the skin and sloughing off of dead cells. If used for a period of time, it seems to plump up and smooth thinning, wrinkled, and sun-damaged skin. It lessens lines and wrinkles, and accelerates the production of new skin cells.

There are problems and side effects that occur with the use of Retin-A, however. Many different adverse reactions have been documented, including skin irritation, redness, and, in many cases, rashes characterized as eczema-like breakouts. People with darker skin may experience dyspigmentation (a lightening, darkening, or mottling of the skin). And although Retin-A is used to help restore the health and appearance of sun-damaged (photo-aged) skin, dermatologists warn that once you become a user of Retin-A, it is more damaging to have any kind of sun exposure and you should *never* go out of the house without using a sunscreen with a very high sun protection factor (SPF).

In an effort to address some of the negative side effects of Retin-A, there has been extensive research aimed at developing a different type of vitamin-A compound that would have significant renewal effects with fewer side effects. Renova, a milder form of Retin-A in a moisturizing base, has been approved by the U.S. Food and Drug Administration (FDA). Like Retin-A, Renova is a prescription drug, and although side effects are less pronounced, they still exist. Another formula has been developed and patented that uses a vitamin-A ester and a process called micellization. This new vitamin-A substance may offer an answer to the irritation problem.

I am happy to say, however, that sun sensitivity and skin irritation are not a problem with my simple technique of epidermabrasion. The youthful appearance of the skin is accomplished simply by ridding the skin of those several top layers of dead, dry skin cells that, when left on the surface, slow down the process of cellular regeneration, leading to the premature formation of lines and wrinkles and preventing fresh young skin cells from rising to the surface.

ALPHA-HYDROXY ACIDS

Another group of so-called miracle ingredients are called alpha-hydroxy acids. These acids too have a reputation for being exfoliating agents (and, interestingly, have been used, in primitive forms, as far back as Cleopatra's time). Alpha-hydroxy acids, however, are not known to cause the serious irritating side effects that are so common with Retin-A. Remember, exfoliation is just another way of saying epidermabrasion, which means sloughing off the dead, dry skin cells that slow down cell renewal and impede moisturizers and nutrient creams from doing their work.

"Everyone seems to be talking about alpha-hydroxy acids lately, but they're not really new—Cleopatra used them in her beauty rituals 2,000 years ago."

The term *alpha-hydroxy acid* can refer to any one of a group of simple, naturally occurring acids. Most of the alpha-hydroxy acids in use today are derived from fruits, milk, and sugar cane and other plants. The important feature of alpha-hydroxy acids is that they have the ability to loosen the bond between the top layers of dead skin cells. Picture this as an ungluing process. Loosening this bond stimulates the body's natural sloughing process, allowing newer, fresher skin cells to emerge, and lessening fine lines, excessive dryness, wrinkles, and sun damage. The use of alpha-hydroxy acids has also been found to reduce discoloration and to even out pigmentation. Several years ago, scientists began to do research using alpha-hydroxy acids on sun-damaged skin. When applied topically, these acids seem to diminish existing sun damage.

Alpha-hydroxy acid (mainly glycolic acid) peels—in which a more highly concentrated alpha-hydroxy acid solution is applied to the skin for a specified period of time to increase the rate of the skin's sloughing process—are a great asset in correcting sun-aging problems. I have found that by utilizing my epidermabrasion and isometric facial exercise technique in combination with products containing medium-level concentrations of alpha-hydroxy acids, it is possible to achieve even more dramatic and effective results. I can truthfully state that I have seen the results of using alpha-hydroxy acids before my very eyes. It has been very exciting to be on this cutting edge of modern skin science, as it has been to witness the visible and immediate improvement in the skin and muscle tone of men and women who have gotten into the habit of doing my very simple routine on a daily basis.

Not only do alpha-hydroxy acids work well on aging skin, they also help oily or acne-prone skin. When dead skin cells build up around hair follicles, they interfere with the natural drainage of the sebaceous (oil-secreting) glands, causing them to clog and fill up. This of course results in acne problems, including pimples, blackheads, and whiteheads. By loosening the bond that glues together the surface layers of dead skin cells, alpha-hydroxy acids release the excessive buildup of these cells and also of toxins embedded in the skin. Like Retin-A, alpha-hydroxy acids help to unblock and cleanse the pores, allowing the skin to rid itself of oils and toxins naturally.

One alpha-hydroxy acid, glycolic acid, which comes from sugar cane, has received a great deal of acclaim. Glycolic acid is the one that dermatologists and licensed estheticians most often use for deeper skin peels and other intensive treatments. However, it has been proven that when glycolic acid is combined with lactic acid in the proper pH balance (below 5), it is equally effective, if not more so. Glycolic acid is also very effective when combined with other alpha-hydroxy acids in skin care products for keeping the skin continually recharged, rejuvenated, smooth, and young-looking.

Lactic acid is an alpha-hydroxy acid that is derived from milk products, specifically sour milk. One of the ancient beauty rituals said to have been used by Cleopatra herself was bathing in milk. (Pretty smart lady, wouldn't you say?) She even had a special tool, called a strygil, to scrape dirt and excess oil off her skin. She was, of course, sloughing off her dry and aging skin cells at the same time.

There are also many legends concerning the use of wine—which contains tartaric acid, another alpha-hydroxy acid—for skin care. In the days of ancient Rome, women would collect the sludge from wine urns and apply it to their faces in the form of a skin pack or facial mask. They would leave it on overnight and it would dissolve the dead, dry skin, leaving a smoother, younger looking skin surface. The same practice was followed by women during the French Revolution. Stories of wine facials have been handed down from generation to generation. I also remember reading stories about a nineteenth-century queen known as Elizabeth of Hungary, who was said to have the most perfect, translucent skin in Europe. I think of her as a royal alchemist. She bathed in the waters of the famous mineral springs of Hungary, and supposedly mixed lemons, violets, roses, and mint leaves with these waters, which were—and still are—known for their health-giving and beautifying properties. She brewed an infusion (an herbal tea), added it to her favorite wine, and applied the mixture to her face—creating a great beauty secret that eventually became known as Hungary water. According to today's skin science, she was actually using a combination of alpha-hydroxy acids. Just remember, the next time you're ready to throw out that old bottle of wine, you might want to splash some of it on your face and see what happens.

Malic acid, which is extracted from apples or bilberries, is also used quite frequently. There are also other, less well known, fruit acids such as pyruvic and gluconic acid. In general, the alpha-hydroxy acids that are more well known are chosen and used for their greater degree of effectiveness.

"The next time you're ready to throw out that old bottle of wine, you might want to splash some of it on your face and see what happens."

Also very widely used is citric acid, another hydroxy acid, which is derived from citrus and other fruits. I have always felt that citrus extracts are wonderful for the skin because they keep the skin's acid mantle (pH balance) at the healthiest level. Also, citrus fruits are loaded with vitamin C and bioflavonoids, especially rutin, which are known to strengthen the tiny capillaries that nourish the skin. History tells us that Cleopatra also used citrus fruits in her beauty rituals. She was said to have massaged sliced-up lemons all over her face, until her skin glowed. (I wonder if she did this before or after the milk bath?) And let me not forget the Duchess of Alba, in Spain, whose beauty was supposedly flawless and ageless, and who was said to have used oranges on her face, throat, and shoulders to prevent aging of the skin and signs of fatigue. The Duchess would apply the pulp of the orange and leave it on for twenty minutes, like a mask. Then she would remove it with water or a mild skin tonic. It is well known that oranges contain a great deal of vitamin C. As we will see in Chapter 6, vitamin C is now also being heralded as one of the most powerful antioxidants and protectors against cellular damage, and is the focus of a great deal of skin care product research and development. Cleopatra and the Duchess of Alba may not have known the scientific explanation for what they were doing, and they might not have realized that they were giving themselves daily mild skin peelings, but they must have been, intuitively, doing something very right, because history tells us that their gorgeous complexions were famous throughout the world.

Another group of acids that have been used for many years are salicylic, benzoic, and buteric acids. They have long been used in over-the-counter acne preparations, and are now being added to other types of products and called beta-hydroxy acids. They are similar to alpha-hydroxy acids in their action, but they have a slightly different chemical structure. Like alpha-hydroxy acids, they have the effect of exfoliating the skin. Many cosmetic companies are now combining alpha- and beta-hydroxy acids in skin care products.

The percentage of alpha- or beta-hydroxy acids present depends on the type of product they are used in, the manufacturer, and the specific formula. For instance, a cleanser does not need as high a percentage because it gets washed off, whereas products like serums, moisturizers, and night treatments should have higher percentages. Alpha-hydroxy acids and/or beta-hydroxy acids can be used in a variety of products, including masks, creams, lotions, scrubs, and cleansers. They are usually used at levels of 5 to 12 percent in serums, creams, and moisturizers for skin rejuvenation, and at higher levels (sometimes even as high as 30 percent) for peels performed by dermatologists and licensed estheticians in skin care salons. Since all licensing of people in the beauty service industry is determined by the particular state you live in, allowable procedures for skin peeling will vary.

CLAY AND MUD MASKS

Clay and mud, applied as masks, are probably the oldest known skin treatments. Legend has it that the beautifying effects of clay and mud were discovered by the royal women of ancient Egypt, who supposedly became jealous of their slave girls when they discovered that the skin on these girls' bodies was more satiny, smooth, and young-looking than their own. Apparently, as the slaves washed clothes in the Nile, they stood deep in the mud of the riverbanks, giving themselves (although unknowingly) an all-over beauty treatment. The mud would remove all the dead, dry, wrinkled skin on their bodies up to the point where they had been immersed, and there would be a line—similar to a suntan line from a bathing suit—where the skin on their bodies changed from very rough to very smooth.

I have always been amazed by the dramatic action of clay and mud (as far as beauty treatments are concerned, they are essentially the same thing). Clay seems to have a natural ability to dissolve

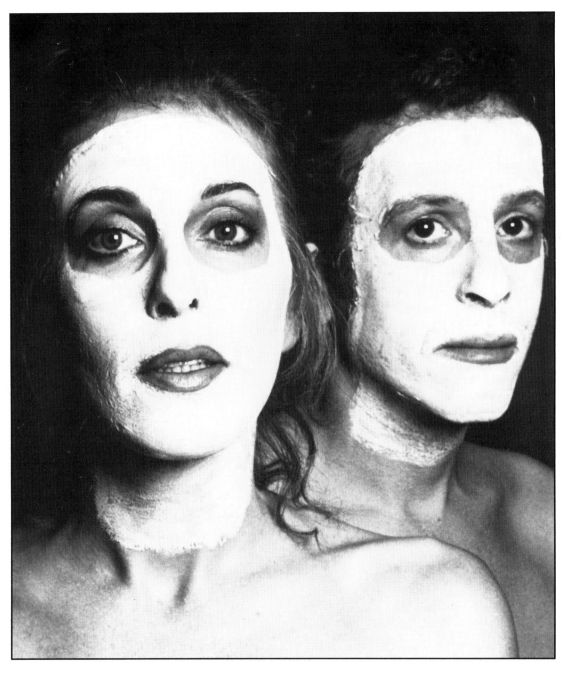

Clay and mud are probably the oldest natural beauty treatments, and they are still among the best.

and absorb dead, dry skin cells. It also has been said to have a magnetic quality that draws toxins from both inside and outside of the body. For this reason, clay is one of my favorite ingredients, and I feel the best facial or body treatment masks are always clay-based. I think you should avoid any peel-off types of masks, because they may peel off more than dirt and grime. Beauty marks may be endangered and tiny hair follicles may be pulled, possibly leading to excess hair growth. No such thing can happen if you use a clay-based mask! Clay is a totally benevolent healing substance full of valuable minerals from the earth.

There are many types of clay from different parts of the world—from the Dead Sea to the Italian Alps, from the Sahara to New Mexico, and on and on. Clay comes in an assortment of colors, from white to red to green, and each type of clay has its own complex of minerals (potassium, magnesium, calcium, etc.), all of which are beneficial and healing. Different types of clay not only dissolve dead, dry skin cells, but help heal many skin irritations as well. Clay also firms and tightens the skin tissue.

I have had the experience of getting up in the morning on a day I was to do a photographic session, having just gotten my menstrual period, and when I looked in the mirror, I saw dark, swollen circles under my eyes. After going through my usual facial regimen, I applied a clay-based mask, waited twenty minutes, and then rinsed it off. Lo and behold, the circles and puffiness were gone! They just seemed to flatten out. This proved to me the great absorbency of the clay-based mask and its power to reduce swelling of skin tissue.

Cleansing and firming masks are quite popular. These usually have a thick consistency and often contain kaolin and bentonite, which are names for different types of clay. As these masks dry, they absorb excess oil, dissolve dirt and dead skin cells, unblock pores, and stimulate circulation. I have also applied clay masks to skin inflammations, burns, and rashes on my body, and found them to be soothing and healing, even when other remedies failed.

For the oily-skinned or acne-prone person, clay masks are an absolute must in skin care, and should be used once or twice a day. At night, a clay mask should be applied to any areas with blemishes and kept on overnight. Clay masks help to clear up breakouts and detoxify skin, with no irritating effects at all. They also help to minimize enlarged pores and refine a bumpy, coarse skin texture. Clay-based products are great for clearing up acne breakouts on the chest, back, and even the arms. Clay has a natural cooling property that soothes complexions that are blotchy, red, or broken out. Not only that, but clay also manages to make the skin feel and look rejuvenated.

For the dry-skinned person, a clay-based mask should be used two to three times a week as part of a stimulating, firming facial that gives a wonderful texture to the skin. Since clay absorbs dead, dry skin cells, there is an automatic renewal of the skin tissue with each use. For the body skin, there are great benefits from the use of this type of mask, if only for the reason that clay and mud are so effective for retexturing and refining the skin. Many of the best health and beauty spas all over the world use different forms of clay and mud to soak the entire body. The treatments are not only tremendously relaxing, but they also remineralize the outer layers of the body skin while giving the skin a baby-soft, firmer, smooth, satiny, and above all younger look and feel.

No matter what your skin type, the use of clay should be included in your plans for lifelong skin rejuvenation. Go out and buy yourself a good clay- or mud-based mask, and discover one of Mother Earth's great beauty gifts.

ENZYMES AND OTHER PEELING SUBSTANCES

Aside from the more publicly acclaimed substances like Retin-A and alpha-hydroxy acids, there are some really great natural enzymes that have a peeling action when used in skin care products. I feel strongly about one called papain, which comes from the papaya fruit and is wonderful for dissolving and peeling away dead, dry skin cells. It is great in masks and scrubs. I have been using papaya for years and have found it to be very good for regenerating and renewing skin tissue. Another enzyme that works well is an extract from the pineapple called bromelain.

One of my favorite ingredients for skin peeling and epidermabrasion is simply salt. Salt has been used for centuries for the purpose of epidermabrading the skin, and it is absolutely great! Once again, we find that history repeats itself; Isadora Duncan, the famous and innovative dancer of the 1920s, was known throughout the world for her gorgeous and satiny skin. She massaged her entire body with salt on a daily basis. Today, it is still the custom of many beauty spas to give their clients salt rubs. A salt rub smooths and purifies the skin, releases toxins, and boosts blood circulation throughout the body. It also generates a tremendous sense of well-being. I recommend using salt in the form of sea salt and granulated sea kelp, because of the presence of additional beneficial minerals derived from the ocean.

"For an invigorating and purifying body treatment, try one of Isadora Duncan's beauty secrets: a salt rub."

There are other substances that can be used for skin peeling, but these are applied only by dermatologists or plastic surgeons. One is trichloroacetic acid; another is called phenolic acid. I repeat, these are used only by physicians, because they are much stronger chemical peels. Generally, people do not need to have this type of peel unless they have very deep scarring or acne-pitted skin. In most cases, a 30-percent solution of glycolic acid will accomplish the desired results.

Throughout this chapter, I have endeavored to make you aware of the greatest new scientific breakthroughs in the field of skin care technology. I have also showed how the great beauties of the past often had the amazing intuition to use basically the same ingredients (albeit in a much more primitive way than modern skin care scientists). I find this very intriguing, and it has certainly helped to make the history of skin care and cosmetics a colorful and romantic voyage that is not only beneficial to learn from but delightful and fun as well.

It seems that in all fields of research, plateaus are reached and maintained for a period of time, and then suddenly tremendous activity occurs and new changes happen very rapidly. Even though I am committed to continually educating myself regarding every new aspect of skin care, I find that at the present time, changes are occurring so rapidly that it takes constant vigilance to keep up with the ongoing developments.

Although I could write chapters on these new peeling agents, I would like to make it clear that although I am in favor of the use of these ingredients, I also believe that all of these things are not a substitute for, but an addition to, my facial exercise and massage technique. They are an extra bonus, definitely *not* a substitute. Skin regeneration is all about epidermibrasion and sanding the skin with friction, to increase circulation, remove dead layers of skin, and bring about a younger and clearer complexion. All of this can be accomplished with a good natural facial scrub. I now feel that the addition of alpha-hydroxy acids in facial products can be very beneficial to the whole process. That is why I am now integrating alpha-hydroxy acids into my natural skin care products. When the skin is epidermabraded before alpha-hydroxy acids are used, this opens the skin up to receiving their benefits, and their effectiveness is increased. In other words, you are accelerating the regeneration process even more than you would if you just used an alpha-hydroxy acid product. The use of great skin care products, along with the exercising and massaging of the facial muscles, is what my technique is all about!

CHAPTER 6

Antioxidants and Free Radicals—
The Good Guys Versus the Bad Guys

There has been much research on which ingredients in skin care products do the best job of moisturizing, nourishing, and protecting the skin. As discussed in Chapter 4, there are treatment creams on the market containing soluble proteins that are used to help the skin achieve a firmer, smoother look and feel. These help build healthy skin tissue. There are also excellent creams containing vitamins, herbs, botanicals, and enzymes that have been shown to have excellent rejuvenating effects on the skin. Another important area of research concerns the use of a group of substances known as antioxidants, which promote the oxygenation of cells.

FREE RADICALS

There are two words that have become more and more a part of public awareness in the last few years: free radicals. As I often say when I am lecturing, free radicals are not necessarily hippies from the sixties. They are highly reactive, unstable atoms or molecules. There are many different types of free radicals, and they form in the body as the result of a number of different processes. Some of them are a byproduct of normal metabolism. Others may be present as a result of the consumption of rancid oils; exposure to smog, automobile exhaust, x-rays, too much sunlight, or chlorine in drinking water; stress; or the basic aging process.

"Free radicals are not hippies from the sixties. They are highly reactive, unstable atoms and molecules that cause degenerative diseases and accelerate aging."

If the body's chemical balance is normal, it may utilize or neutralize free radicals as quickly as they are formed, and they will not do any harm. But in our modern, industrialized environment we are continually being bombarded with free radicals. If there are more free radicals than the body can cope with, they become toxic and can become involved in causing degenerative diseases. Free radicals also accelerate the aging process of the entire body, including, obviously, the skin. They attack healthy skin cell membranes, the skin's collagen and elastin protein fibers, and all the genetic material inside the living cells. This causes cellular damage and leads to degenerative diseases and aging.

ANTIOXIDANTS

The greatest defense we know of against free radical damage is a class of substances known as antioxidants, which have the ability to keep free radicals from reacting in dangerous ways in the body. Specifically, they can interrupt or block oxidation reactions involving free radicals. Oxidation is a term for any chemical reaction involving oxygen. Many oxidation reactions involve some kind of degeneration or spoilage. When iron rusts, vegetable oil becomes rancid, apples turn brown, or silver tarnishes, oxidation is taking place. Antioxidants block the oxidation process. As a result, healthy cells remain unharmed.

Since free radicals attack the DNA and RNA in the cell nuclei, causing cellular damage, it is important that antioxidants be taken and used to fight the formation—and aid in the destruction—of these free radicals. Antioxidants can be taken internally, in the form of nutritional supplements, to benefit the entire body. They can also be applied externally, to benefit the skin. Antioxidants occur in a variety of different substances, including certain vitamins, minerals, botanicals (plant extracts), enzymes, and trace elements.

Superoxide Dismutase

Superoxide dismutase (also known by its abbreviation, SOD) is an antioxidant that has shown excellent benefits in fighting free radical damage. SOD is a nutrient enzyme. It can be derived from animal sources, but it is now available as a natural derivative of yeast. It also occurs naturally in such foods as broccoli, Brussels sprouts, cabbage, and many other green plants.

By its action as an antioxidant, SOD increases the oxygenation of skin cells and helps to protect them from toxins. It also helps to stimulate collagen production. Research on SOD has shown it to be effective in slowing the progression of aging, cancer, arthritis, and muscular dystrophy. In other words, this enzyme seems to be able to control cellular degeneration and boost the immune system as a whole, thereby stimulating healthy cell regeneration on both the inside and the outside of the body.

Selenium

Another highly acclaimed antioxidant is the trace element selenium. Selenium has been shown to limit damage to cells caused by oxidation, therefore fighting disease and aging. It has been used successfully to strengthen the immune system and also to lower the rate of skin cancer.

Selenium works synergistically with vitamin E. Studies have shown that a combination of selenium, vitamin E, and vitamin C protects lung tissue from damage and disease. The tissues of other organs should benefit as well—and remember, the skin is the body's largest organ.

Four Important Vitamins

Although vitamins have been used in skin care preparations for many, many years, skin care science is rediscovering and retesting the efficacy of these vitamins on a whole new level. After reviewing the literature and interviewing biochemists, I have come up with my own recommendation. It occurred to me that after you apply the alpha-hydroxy acid product of your choice, your skin is able to rid itself of that buildup of dry, dead skin cells (remember that epidermabrading the skin with a good facial scrub before applying the alpha-hydroxy acid product doubles the beneficial results). After this peeling-away process, the skin is more receptive than ever to the benefits of nutrients.

Vitamin E

There is now documented and unanimous agreement in the scientific community concerning the topical application of skin care products containing significant amounts of vitamin E. For years, vitamin E has been known to inhibit spoilage and rancidity, and has even been included as a preservative in skin care products. Lester Packer, professor of molecular and cell biology at the University of California, Berkeley, and one of the nation's leading experts on vitamin E, says, "Unlike other vitamins, the topical application of vitamin E acetate and vitamin E linoleate most often used in skin care creams is the one that most effectively penetrates the skin. It is absorbed by cell membranes and forms a protective antioxidant defense against free radical damage, including sun damage. It is also a natural moisturizer that prevents evaporation of water from the skin cells." For years, vitamin E has been used to soothe and repair skin tissue, scar tissue, and inflammation, especially when the skin has suffered burns—particularly sunburn. It has also been shown to help minimize stretch marks caused by weight gain or pregnancy.

When vitamin E is combined with vitamin C, these two vitamins form one of the most potent antioxidant weapons against free radical damage. It has always been difficult to combine these two vitamins, because they are not normally compatible (vitamin C is water-soluble; vitamin E is oil-soluble). Through methods of encapsulation, however, skin care science has now found ways to deliver these vitamins together into the skin cells. Biochemist John Trevithick and his colleagues at the University of Wisconsin found that when vitamin E was applied to skin after exposure to sun or ultraviolet radiation, the amount of swelling, redness, and sensitivity was dramatically reduced—as much as 50 percent in some cases.

When looking for a skin care or cosmetic product that is a good source of vitamin E, be aware that this nutrient can appear on labels in a variety of ways. It may be called simply vitamin E, or it may be called any one of the following: tocopherol acetate, tocopherol linoleate, alpha tocopherol, or vitamin-E acetate. Scientists also agree that for a cream, lotion, or oil to be effective, there should be a substantial percentage of vitamin E in it. In other words, if vitamin E is the last ingredient listed on the package, it won't do you much good. My personal recommendation would be to use a special cream, lotion, or oil with at least 10,000 international units of vitamin E, even if other creams or lotions you use contain lesser amounts.

Vitamin A

The vitamin-A derivative known as retinyl palmitate (not to be confused with Retin-A, which is another derivative of vitamin A; see Chapter 5) is known as a skin normalizer. Retinyl palmitate has not been as widely used in skin care as vitamin E because skin care scientists believed that it could not penetrate the skin as well. However, recent studies have shown that, if formulated properly and used at the right levels, vitamin A can indeed penetrate and impart very important benefits, such as increasing the skin's elasticity; smoothing and normalizing dry, parched skin; and reversing ultraviolet or sun damage. It also gives great antioxidant protection. Vitamin A is known to be a powerful antioxidant, and it is the subject of research and development aimed at enabling it to penetrate effectively into the skin. Vitamin A may appear on product labels as vitamin A, or as retinyl palmitate (noted above), beta-carotene, tretinoin, or retinoic acid.

Vitamin C

Many people call vitamin C the supreme nutrient, because its performance and action are so versatile. Indeed, a deficiency of this vitamin can produce maladies ranging from scurvy to increased susceptibility to all kinds of infection and disease. One obvious benefit of having a sufficient amount of vitamin C in your system is that it can raise the ability of the immune system to withstand and fight off many different ailments. By now, vitamin C has become one of the most basic and universal family remedies—almost better than chicken soup!

Vitamin C also, of course, is a very powerful antioxidant. I have always believed that vitamin C has been a "diamond in the rough" in terms of topical application. Because of my studies of nutrition, I knew that this vitamin has proven to be essential for the formation and strengthening of collagen fibers; scientific research has shown that vitamin C stimulates and actually speeds up the regeneration of collagen-producing fibroblasts that make up the capillaries and membranes of the skin tissue. Knowing this, I always felt that vitamin C would be incredibly beneficial if applied directly to the skin. The problem here has been—and I do mean "has been"—that unlike vitamins E and A, which are oil-soluble and are able to hold their poten-

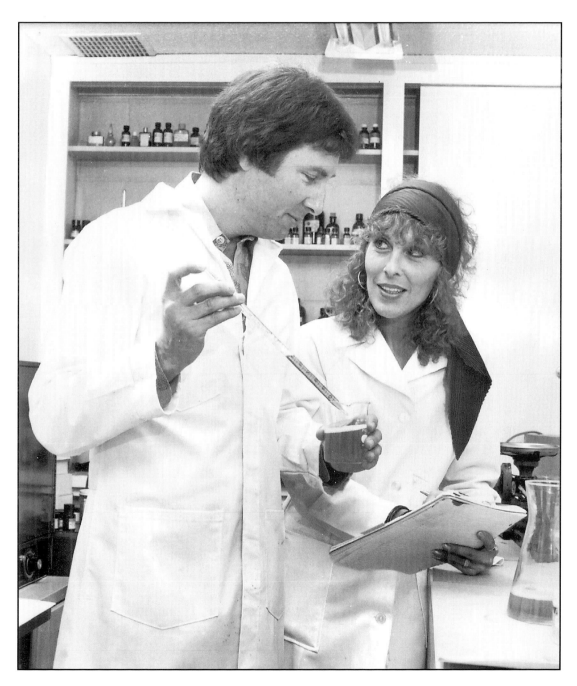

Modern skin care science is constantly learning more
and more about using vitamins, minerals, botanicals,
and other natural ingredients in skin care products.

"For years, vitamin C has been considered one of the most basic and universal family remedies— almost better than chicken soup! Now we know it's great for your skin, too."

cy in skin care products, vitamin C is water-soluble and loses its potency through evaporation. For my own personal use and the use of my students and clients, I devised my own solution, which is to buy a jar of natural buffered vitamin-C powder and mix it into my scrubs, masks, creams, and cleansing products. The important thing to remember is that you have to take a portion of the skin care product from the jar, pour it into a dish, add approximately one-eighth teaspoon of vitamin-C powder per one teaspoon of product, and mix and apply the product immediately. You can't save it until the next day or the potency will go bye-bye. This extra effort is a small price to pay for the results you will experience. I have seen a definite new firmness and strength in my own skin tissue, as well as in the skin of clients of mine who have done this. After all, my whole technique and philosophy is about the strengthening of both muscles and overlying skin tissue. I have even had tiny broken capillaries right under the surface of the skin disappear with this treatment.

I always felt, however, that there had to be a way of making the addition of vitamin C to skin care products work. And the great news is that finally there has been a major breakthrough in the technology of delivering vitamin C to the skin without it losing its potency. This came about in the field of liposome research. It is now possible to encapsulate vitamin C so that its potency is preserved until it penetrates the layers of the skin to impart its rewards (see pages 41–44 for a detailed explanation of liposomes and how they work). The wonderful thing about these new delivery systems is that they are formulated with natural materials, not harsh chemicals.

Because vitamin C exists in citrus fruits, which are the source of citric acid (one of the hydroxy acids), you may think it would be redundant to use vitamin C in addition to citric acid. However, in my years of studying nutrition and biochemistry, I have learned that there are many constituents that make up a total vitamin complex. Remember the example of the different derivatives of vitamin A, including Retin-A, retinyl palmitate, and beta-carotene. These are all different aspects of the same vitamin. Vitamin C has within its natural complex several components, such as the bioflavonoids rutin and hesperidin, that are essential and very beneficial, and that cannot be obtained when vitamin C is presented in the form of ascorbic acid alone. Nature is quite miraculous, and the duplication of any naturally occurring substance is as difficult to achieve as the duplication of the DNA codes in our bodies would be. In any case, using pure, natural vitamin C complex, whether in powder form or in the new encapsulated liposomes, will ensure that you are really getting the utmost benefit of this vitamin complex. Vitamin C may be listed on product labels as any one of a number of different compounds, including ascorbic acid, ascorbyl palmitate, and ester-C.

The B Vitamins

Pantothenic acid—also called panthenol, d-panthenol, and pro-vitamin B_5—is a member of the vitamin-B complex group that is present in all living cells. It is the most effective B vitamin for skin care and hair care. It is used very often in both skin and hair care because it has been proved to penetrate skin and hair tissue rapidly and to provide lasting moisturization. It has also been shown to stimulate the regeneration and repair of skin tissue. Niacinamide, a form of another member of the vitamin-B complex (vitamin B_3, or niacin), is also beneficial.

Botanicals

In addition to vitamins, minerals, and enzymes, there are also botanicals that have antioxidant properties. Suma, which is rich in the antioxidant trace element germanium, is grown in the Brazilian rain forest. It is known for its detoxifying, healing, oxygenating, and immune-strengthening properties. Suma also makes a great tea, which I have found to relieve everything from cold and flu symptoms

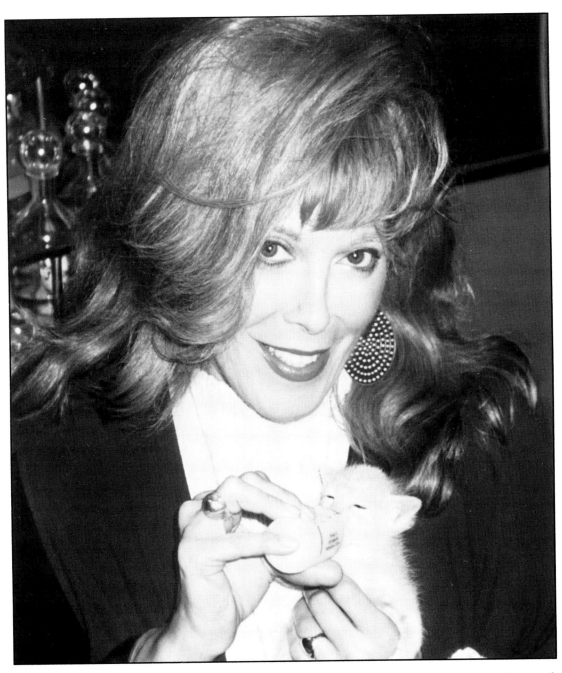

I am very dedicated to animal rights. Here I am with one of the many baby animals I have played Mommy to.

to stomach cramps and fatigue. Some of the richest antioxidant plant treasures are grown in the world's rain forests. This is yet another reason that the destruction of these forests is a horrible tragedy for mankind.

Long before synthetic formulations were developed, the natives of rain forest regions were using their own botanical plants, herbs, and oils to cleanse, purify, moisturize, nourish, and heal their skin, as well as to cure their physical ailments (these special botanicals are denoted by an asterisk in Appendix I, A Glossary of Nature's Bountiful Gifts). Like so many other people in past centuries, these people knew—way before the scientific community started doing research—that these rain forest botanicals held a treasure trove of therapeutic benefits. After all, the inhabitants of the rain forests were using these plant substances every day of their lives, for centuries. Only in the last few years has modern skin care research seriously investigated the properties and benefits inherent in these plants.

We now know that the climate and environment of rain forest areas make possible the existence of unique and medicinal substances not found in other environments. Harnessing the remarkable powers in these botanicals has been very exciting work.

Another powerful antioxidant is Pycnogenol (pronounced pik-NAH-ji-nol), which is derived from the bark of a pine tree called the anneda pine tree. This plant is known to have been used as a medicinal tea by North American natives in the region of what is now Quebec, Canada, as far back as the year 1535. It has been said that they gave this tea to French explorers and cured them of scurvy, a vitamin-C deficiency disease that was very common among sailors on long ocean voyages in those days. Some research has shown that Pycnogenol is a super antioxidant, possibly as much as fifty times more powerful than vitamin E. It has been shown to help retard aging, stimulate blood circulation, and improve vision, and possibly to reduce the risk of cancer, heart disease, and a variety of other health problems.

Other botanicals that have strong antioxidant properties include ginseng, ginkgo biloba, chamomile, calendula, goldenseal, echinacea, milk thistle, and many more. The study of these botanicals, vitamins, minerals, enzymes, and trace elements that are great antioxidants is fascinating. All of these are ingredients to look for when you are buying any kind of skin care product.

It is really quite wonderful and amazing to realize that the answers and remedies for many of our human ailments can be found in nature's bountiful gifts from the sea and the earth. As the earth's inhabitants, we should be the guardians of its treasures, and of human and animal rights. Let's celebrate the earth as we celebrate our lives!

CHAPTER 7

The Sun—Friend or Foe?

The sun has so many wonderful benefits for our bodies and souls. Poems, paintings, and songs have been created in homage to its glories. The sun warms us, gives us vitamin D just by shining on us, and makes us feel good all over. Unfortunately, however, we now know that exposure to the sun's rays is also the most prevalent cause of the aging of the skin. The sun's ultraviolet and infrared rays are responsible for many of the skin-related problems associated with aging, such as age spots, dyspigmentation, deep lines and wrinkles, and, worst of all, skin cancer. According to biomedical researcher Peter Pugliese, M.D., "At least ninety percent of the problems related to aging skin are the result of sun exposure."[1]

There are two different types of ultraviolet rays, known as UVA and UVB rays, that can cause skin damage. UVB rays are the "burning" rays, and are present in the greatest concentrations in the middle of the day and in the summer. UVA rays, in contrast, do not usually cause the same type of sunburn, but they do cause sun damage.

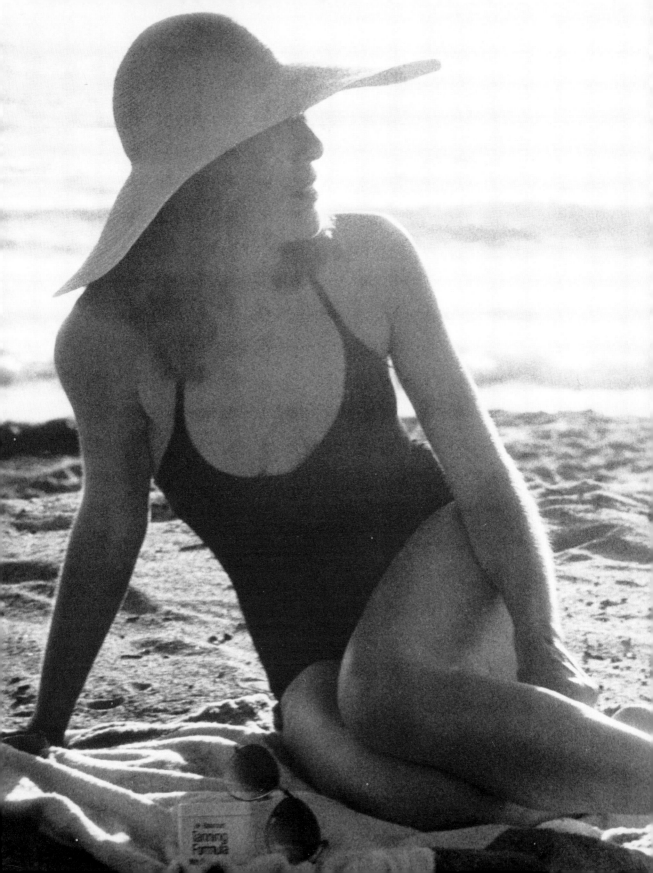

Also, they are present all day long and do not diminish in the winter. I made up a little rhyme that helps to explain the difference between UVA and UVB rays: "UVA lasts all day; UVB from ten to three."

In the past, it was believed that UVB rays posed a greater hazard than UVA, but research now shows that long-term damage caused by UVA rays is also a factor in premature aging and even skin cancer. So even though UVA rays may exist at times of the day or in areas of the world where the sun may not be shining and hot, they can still be very, very dangerous and damaging to the skin. "Sunlight reflects on your skin while you are walking down the street, biking, and even driving in a car. Since UVA rays can even penetrate through glass windows, they account for more than 70 percent of sun damage," says Albert Clemens, M.D., of the Department of Dermatology at the University of Pennsylvania. The degree of UV exposure is also influenced by environmental factors such as altitude, latitude, and the thickness of the ozone layer. The thinner the ozone layer, the more ultraviolet rays reach the earth. If you are serious about retarding the aging of your skin, you must take steps to protect your skin correctly from sun damage all year round.

THE TRUTH ABOUT TANNING

When the skin is exposed to the sunlight, it attempts to use its natural defenses to prevent burning. The skin contains a protective dark pigment called melanin. When the skin is exposed to the sun, the melanin rises to the surface to absorb the sun's ultraviolet rays. This is what causes the phenomenon we know as tanning. In other words, melanin is the skin's protective mechanism against burning; a suntan is the way it manifests itself.

Darker skinned people have more protective melanin in their skin than lighter skinned people do, so they can take more sun exposure before any damaging effects occur. However, even the darkest skin will eventually burn, and over time it will become leathery and uneven in coloration as a result of too much sun. Fair-skinned people, especially blonds and redheads, have much less melanin in their skin and therefore have much less natural defense against the sun.

One way of thinking about it is that you are born with a particular skin color, and when you get a dark tan you are really changing the cellular structure of your skin. The texture thickens and becomes leathery and wrinkled as the skin's natural elasticity starts to break down. Despite the popular concept of the "healthy tan," a suntan is actually a not-so-healthy thing to do to your skin.

A term that is frequently used to describe skin that has been prematurely aged by sun exposure is "photo-aged." Photo-aging is caused by excessive exposure to sunlight, especially over the long term, which adversely affects all of the skin's structural elements. With repeated exposure, a cumulative and continuous breakdown of the skin's elastin and collagen fibers occurs. The sad thing is that this damage may become apparent only years later. The signs of photo-aged skin are deep wrinkles, yellowing, enlarged pores, blotchiness, a coarse and rough texture, a leathery look, and, once again, the loss of elasticity (a basic sagginess). Also, and very sadly, photo-aged skin is more vulnerable to melanomas and other cancerous and pre-cancerous tumors. Now that so many members of the "baby boom" generation are over forty, they are paying the price for all those past suntans they once thought looked so healthy and attractive—since, I repeat, the effects are cumulative.

As far as tanning booths are concerned, the radiation they emit carries all the risks of real sunlight and long-term exposure. Even though the advertising sometimes tries to lead you to believe otherwise, the rays used in tanning parlors are still a cause of skin cancer and premature aging, and even cataracts of the eyes—just like the real thing. In addition, in many places tanning parlors are unregulated, and allow customers access to tanning beds without supervision or eye protection.

"'UVA lasts all day; UVB from ten to three'—and to avoid premature aging, you have to protect your skin from both types of ultraviolet rays."

SUN PROTECTION

What can we do to protect ourselves against sun damage? Fortunately, there are now protective defenses that really work. The initials SPF stand for *sun protection factor*. SPF numbers indicate how many times longer than normal a sunscreen makes it possible to stay in the sun without burning. So, for example, using a product with an SPF of 8 would theoretically make it possible for you to be in the sun eight times longer than you normally could without burning (although I personally would not recommend that anyone ever do more than half an hour of sunbathing).

Thanks to modern skin science, sunscreens and sun blocks are now available in a wide range of SPFs to help prevent the development of photo-aged wrinkles. In fact, a whole numbers game is going on in the skin care industry regarding SPFs and sun creams. Everywhere you go, you see on the shelves sunscreens and sun blocks ranging from SPF 2 to SPF 50. Two important words to look for when selecting sunscreen or sun block products are *broad spectrum*. This means protection against all ultraviolet rays, both UVA and UVB. Also, it is important to understand the difference between a sunscreen and a sun block. Sunscreens range from SPF 2 to SPF 15, and screen out a certain percentage of harmful rays. Anything SPF 15 or over is supposed to completely block out all harmful rays and is therefore called a sun block. A sunscreen with an SPF of 15 or more supposedly will block more than 93 percent of the sun's damaging rays, and make it possible to be out in the sun fifteen times longer than you normally could before your skin will suffer sun damage. Theoretically, a product with an SPF of 15 is supposed to provide adequate all-day protection, as long as it remains on the skin. I personally do not believe, however, that a sun protection product will remain on the skin without continual reapplication throughout the day, because of swimming, perspiration, etc. I also do not believe that science has as yet found any complete protection against the more cumulative and damaging UVA rays.

The state of the art in sun protection is continually changing and improving, as researchers are always looking into the creation of better sunscreens and sun blocks. The latest breakthrough in sun shields is the use of micronized powders made from titanium dioxide and zinc oxide. At one time, these protective substances were available only in the form of greasy white ointments—the stuff you would see on lifeguards' noses. But they can now be crushed into a sheer powder form and suspended in hypoallergenic creams or even transparent sun protection products.

Titanium dioxide, unlike traditional chemical sunscreens, reflects light rather than absorbing it. It also blocks out infrared light, an additional benefit to sun-sensitive skin. These fine particles, often listed on product labels as TiO_2, have made it possible for skin care product manufacturers to formulate highly effective broad-spectrum sunscreens that can be used safely at higher levels not only in sun care products, but in skin care products and cosmetics as well. Makeup foundation always contains titanium dioxide, which is why it is so protective for the skin.

Another approach now being experimented with involves the use of melanin as a sunscreen for extra UVA protection. As I mentioned earlier, melanin is the natural protective pigment in the skin. It is melanin, which is more prevalent in darker complexions, that makes darker skinned people less susceptible to sunburn. Melanin could conceivably be blended with other sunscreens and sun blocks to give even more protection against both UVA and UVB Rays. Keep looking for new innovations, as the science of sun protection is constantly growing and evolving.

In addition to sunscreens, the best of the sun care products contain other beneficial ingredients, such as vitamins E, A, and C; rain forest botanicals like suma, kukui nut, agave, copaiba, and babassu; and other soothing ingredients, such as aloe vera, cocoa butter, Brazil nut oil, chamomile, shea butter, and squalane. Research has been going on for many years regarding vitamin C. One recent study on the use of vitamin C substantiates its use as a nontoxic and long-lasting sunscreen. In addition, any ingredient that is also an antioxidant (see Chapter 6) will help the skin to combat free radicals that form as a result of sun exposure.

What about self-tanning products? There are many products on the market today that can give you a suntanned look—without the sun. They all contain one key ingredient, called dihydroxyacetone (DHA). This ingredient affects the dead cells on the top layer of the skin, turning them a suntanned color. As the skin sheds, either through its own natural process or through epidermabrasion, the color disappears, usually in three days to one week. I have been told by dermatologists and skin care experts that these products seem to have no harmful effects. For people who just can't give up on the idea of having a tan, I feel that the use of this type of product is a lot safer than lying out in the sun to get a real one.

Any way you cut it, sun protection is a very, very serious subject, and "safe sun" is just as important as any other safety topic in this day and age. Be sure to keep yourself protected, and reapply sun protection products throughout the day to every exposed part of your body (don't forget your lips!). See Table 7.1 for my sun care recommendations.

For myself, I am quite happy to have my medium-fair complexion—and many fewer lines than my sun-worshiping friends. Many of them are now coming to me for advice on how to reverse their sun damage. If you have significant sun damage, I advise the use of medically prescribed Retin-A as well as skin care products containing alpha-hydroxy acids and antioxidants—and, of course, my own basic technique! But my slogan is "Avert the danger and the disaster before it has the chance to happen." After all, we were all born with the color skin we were supposed to have. Your skin will look so beautiful if you follow the guidelines in this book, your own rosy glow will make a suntan seem quite unnecessary and even undesirable.

Table 7.1 Sun Care Recommendations

This table lists sun care products and precautions that are appropriate for different skin types. If you are unsure about what type of skin you have, see Know Your Skin Type on page 34. Whatever your skin type, always remember that your skin is exposed to the sun's rays anytime you are outdoors—no matter what you are doing, what season or time of day it is, or what the weather is like—so sun protection is a necessity every day.

SKIN TYPE	SUN CARE RECOMMENDATIONS	
	SUN CARE FOR BODY AND FACE	LIP PROTECTION AND MOISTURIZING
Normal and Combination Skin	Good sunscreen or sun block cream or lotion with an SPF of at least 6–15, applied before and during all outdoor activities (every day). Sunscreen can and should be used under moisturizer or makeup.	Moisturizing lip balm with sunscreen, worn either under lipstick or alone (every day).
Dry, Very Dry, and Aging Skin	Good sunscreen or sun block cream or lotion with an SPF 15 or over, applied before and during all outdoor activities (every day). Sunscreen can and should be used under moisturizer or makeup. Look for a formula with one or more of the excellent moisturizing ingredients mentioned in this chapter (see page 81). Allow very little direct sun exposure; wear a hat when outdoors.	Moisturizing lip balm with sunscreen, worn either under lipstick or alone (every day).
Oily or Acne-Prone Skin	Good sunscreen or sun block cream or lotion with an SPF of at least 6–15, applied before and during all outdoor activities (every day). Sunscreen can and should be used under moisturizer or makeup. Choose an oil-free, non-comedogenic (non-pore-clogging) formula. Be careful not to overdo sun exposure.	Moisturizing lip balm with sunscreen, worn either under lipstick or alone (every day).
Sensitive Skin	Good sunscreen or sun block cream or lotion with an SPF 15, applied before and during all outdoor activities (every day). Sunscreen can and should be used under moisturizer or makeup. Look for a formula with special soothing ingredients like chamomile, aloe vera, and vitamin E. Allow no direct sun exposure, especially if you have fair skin.	Moisturizing lip balm with sunscreen, worn either under lipstick or alone (every day).

CHAPTER 8

Skin Fitness
for the Body Beautiful

I think you would agree that we are living in a day and age in which there is an extreme emphasis on all-over body fitness. Being out of shape is definitely *not* in. Every time you turn on the TV, you see someone in a leotard (or practically nude) who is either dieting, exercising, massaging, cleansing, or lubricating his or her body beautiful. Personally, I believe that you can make this trend work for you on a very positive level if you choose to. As I said at the beginning of this book, you do not have to look or feel "over the hill" at any age.

EXERCISE FOR A HEALTHY, HAPPY BODY

Even though I started taking dance classes at an early age, it took me years to get over my resistance to following a really disciplined exercise regime. Am I ever glad that I finally broke through the resistance! My body is in better shape now than when I was sixteen, and I feel better about my body now than I did then. A long time ago, my dear friend and body coach, Bill Landrum, told me that the body actually starts to miss the exercise when it doesn't get its fill. I didn't believe him at the time, but I do now. Bill, who is a talented dancer and choreographer, knows this from the experience of working on himself and with other people. He says that getting regular exercise is like waking up your body. Once you have taken the big step and awakened your body to a new level of strength and vitality, it really doesn't want to go back to sleep. This transition may not happen overnight, because there's that little voice from the past, saying, "I don't want to!" "I'm too tired," "I'm too busy," and so on. After a while, however, you'll find that the more you follow a disciplined exercise routine, the more your body will crave doing it and ask you to keep up the work.

A shot from my video. Regular exercise is absolutely essential for a healthy, "wide-awake" body.

EPIDERMABRASION FOR BODY SKIN

Just as exercise is important for both your face and your body, so the principle of epidermabrasion applies to your body skin as well as to your facial skin. Get a back brush with a long handle (one that feels comfortable) and every time you shower or bathe, massage your entire body—your legs, arms, elbows, back, and chest. If you are a woman, encircle your breast area. Always stroke toward your heart—upward from your feet; downward from your arms. This is important for encouraging lymphatic drainage, stimulating the nerve endings in the skin, and improving all-over muscle tone and cell renewal.

As with your face, let your own skin sensitivity be your guide, and as your skin becomes accustomed to the brush massage, buy a rougher brush. There is nothing wrong with getting out of the shower after a vigorous massage with a very rosy body. It just means that the blood is coming to skin's surface, rejuvenating all the skin tissue and giving all-over healthy circulation. It is also important for helping to break down cellulite (more about that later in this chapter).

Epidermabrading and massaging your body skin should always be the other half of exercising your body's muscles, just as it is for your face. After your dance or yoga class, your tennis game, or whatever type of body exercise you choose, when you are ready to jump into the shower or bath, take that rough brush with you. A good abrasive body scrub can be used for this purpose. I have developed a special body scrub containing seeds, mint leaves, herbs, and marine botanicals that are known to detoxify and rejuvenate the entire body skin. A body scrub can be rubbed on dry skin before a shower or bath; as the grainy scrub is massaged into the body skin, dead, dry surface skin cells are sloughed off and all-over circulation is improved.

Another shot from my video. It can take time to get into the exercise habit, but the results are worth it!

The scrub is then rinsed off in the shower, leaving the skin satiny, invigorated, and glowing. You can use the rough brush for even greater sloughing and stimulation before rinsing off the body scrub.

You can also use the body scrub while you shower. I pour body scrub onto a wet washcloth to massage my entire body; I find that the combination of the body scrub and the wet washcloth makes application easier and provides for better overall coverage. It can be hard to find products that are designed specifically for epidermabrading the body skin, but they are there, and if you find one that looks interesting, by all means try it. After your shower, towel dry with a nice rough towel—not the soft velour type. Those are pretty, but they do nothing for body circulation.

For extra-oily body skin or skin that tends to break out in areas like the upper chest and back, you can apply a clay or mud mask to the affected areas after the scrubbing, showering, and toweling dry. Leave the mask on overnight—every night, if possible—to absorb toxins and excess oil, and it will surely help clear up the body skin. I have found it to be very good for helping to heal abrasions. Clay and mud masks are good for many things. For instance, body massage specialists are now using clay and mud masks on the upper arms and thighs to help tighten, firm, and reestablish skin tone after weight loss. This technique is used in conjunction with exercise. If you would like to try this, I suggest applying a body firm-up mask and leaving it on for twenty minutes two or three times a week. I am also in favor of using saunas, steam baths, thalassotherapy (ocean spray massages), mud baths, and massage, all of which help circulation while relaxing the mind and body. You can lead me to the nearest sauna or Jacuzzi any day. I love it.

Remember a very important point. After your body is scrubbed, steamed, bathed, and toweled dry, it is in need of (and more receptive to) the benefits of a body moisturizer or body oil. There are many good ones on the market. The best are pH-balanced and contain some of the same great and scientifically advanced skin nutrients discussed in Chapter 4. Massage your body with moisturizer from tip to toe and get ready for a new surge of radiant energy. It is your body saying, "Thank you!"

"There's nothing wrong with getting out of the shower after a vigorous massage with a very rosy body. It just means you've increased the blood circulation to the skin's surface."

FINDING CLUES TO THE MYSTERY OF CELLULITE

Ah, the wonders of the bulge-busting, ripple-relieving (oh-so-simple) solutions of thalassotherapy, pulsing electrodes, cellulolipolisis, electric acupuncture, and all the other multi-syllable tongue twisters! I want to talk about the problem of cellulite, but I also want to make sure you understand that everything I am about to say is simply an extension of great body care. It applies to all of us, men as well as women.

Whether we have experienced the problem personally or not, most of us know that the look of cellulite is that not-so-pretty picture of a very, very old overstuffed couch that has been sat on for years. Cellulite is that lumpy, bumpy, plumpy—and not a bit lovely—dimpled-looking skin that appears in areas of the body where excess fat is normally stored. Basically, cellulite forms when waste material from the cells collects in and around the fatty layers beneath the skin. As this waste starts piling up, it forms layers, the skin tissues swell up, and the skin begins to bulge.

Nearly all of the experts on cellulite say that these pockets of fat deposits condense and rise high up into the skin tissue. This is what causes that puckered-up cottage-cheese or orange-peel appearance. Plastic surgeon Peter Fodor, M.D., says, "The mattress look results when fat bulges up around the bands of connective tissue that tie it down to the muscles."[1]

Other experts in the field agree that a problem with the lymphatic system is the primary cause of cellulite. In a healthy body, the blood delivers oxygen to the cells, and the lymphatic and blood flow remove wastes, toxins, and metabolic byproducts from the cells. But if the lymphatic system is clogged, then the toxic waste material cannot be eliminated from the blood. This type of congestion or clogging is basically a buildup of these uneliminated toxins.

Cellulite is not the same as ordinary fat. This is obvious because even very thin people can still fall victim to this culprit. Some people do seem to have more of a genetic tendency to develop cellulite than others, and women are more likely to develop it than men. Certain elements of lifestyle—including a lack of exercise, poor posture, hormonal imbalances, too-shallow breathing, poor diet, and too little fluid intake—also appear to contribute to the formation of cellulite, probably because they contribute to a blocked lymphatic system and, all in all, decreased blood circulation and a sluggish metabolism. But the good news is that there *are* some known methods to minimize cellulite, if not to completely rid yourself of it.

As I have been stating throughout this book, a healthy and active circulatory system is one of the great keys to a youthful body, inside and out. It almost goes without saying that the number-one essential for beating cellulite is regular exercise. This automatically increases circulation and the supply of oxygen to the cells. The second most widely used method of dealing with this problem is correct and specific massage. Massage increases circulation of the blood and lymphatic fluid, thereby reducing blockage and restoring balance to the entire system. Also, kneading an area with cellulite (much as you would knead bread dough) helps to release the toxins, water, and fatty substances that have built up and become trapped in the connective fibers underlying the skin, causing them to squeeze together and become hard and irritated, making the surrounding tissue lose its elasticity and the awful lumpy, orange-peel sight of cellulite start to appear.

I feel a good time to massage your body with a good brush, and to do your kneading, is while you are in the shower. Soon it will become a habit, and you will not want to leave the shower until you have finished working on your body. I even do certain stretching and breathing exercises every day while I'm in the shower; it has become a way of energizing myself for the whole day. Remember, always massage in the direction of your heart. I also recommend that you use your body scrub with a wet washcloth when massaging and kneading your body. Many experts promote dry-brushing with a loofa, ayate cloth, or mitt to massage the body, but I prefer to do it with a rough brush and/or a washcloth with body scrub on it while I'm in the shower. I do a second, dry-brushing massage with the rough-towel technique, discussed earlier in this chapter, while drying myself off after showering.

So, my friends, you no longer have to feel unloved or unneeded, because now you can love and knead yourself! That should definitely help your self-esteem, along with giving you a sensuous and smooth body skin.

Finally, let me not omit the most obvious and universal of all, which is all-over body massage utilizing body creams, oils, or lotions formulated especially for massage. There are certain essential oils and herbs that are really great in a massage formula, including sea algae (and other extracts from the sea), ginseng, eucalyptus, rosemary, juniper, poppy seed, peppermint, capsicum (also known as cayenne or red pepper), spearmint, cypress, orange rind, lemon, camphor, and ivy. I especially love using capsicum in a massage formula to help warm up the muscles and get more blood circulation going.

Plant extracts from the sea are now being used more than any other plant extracts for cellulite problems. Cellulite specialists say that these sea-derived ingredients work the best to release the trapped toxins, excess fat, and water that are stored in these problem areas. They also have a lot of valuable minerals, such as magnesium, potassium, and calcium, plus sea salt, all of which really help purify the body skin. I can't imagine anything more exhilarating than standing in the ocean and getting a seawater hydro-massage. If you are lucky enough to live near an ocean, you can stand in the water so that the waves break against your cellulite areas. Keep in mind that sea kelp, sea algae, sea salt, spirulina, and seaweed all come from the same place. You'll get a remineralizing salt rub and anti-cellulite ocean massage all at the same time! You can also simply lie down on the sand by the water's edge and feel the massage and exfoliating effects of the sand with the ocean's spray and waves—nature's very own spa right on the beach! Sometimes the best things in life can be free. The same type of treatment offered by spa professionals—but definitely not for free—is called *thalassotherapy* (from the Greek *thalassa*, meaning "sea").

Body Care Tips for Pregnancy

Just a few words to you ladies in waiting to remind you that while your body is in the process of changing its size, it is vitally important that you stay on a regimen of muscle-toning and circulation-boosting for both your face and your body. The more consistent you are while you are pregnant, the less of an overhaul you will have to deal with after the stork arrives.

There are many good exercise programs designed for the pregnant woman available from many sources, and I recommend that you follow one. And whatever exercise program you choose, it is most important to do your exercises in conjunction with the epidermabrasion technique described in these pages. This will increase your overall circulation and the vitality of your entire body skin, and will also help to alleviate the pain of aching and tired muscles. Most pregnant women say that keeping their feet raised on pillows and getting frequent foot massages from partners or good friends alleviates a lot of the fatigue caused by carrying so much extra weight.

A great tip to help prevent stretch marks from forming is this: Every single day, without fail, massage your tummy, hips, and thighs with a good body moisturizer or cream containing vitamin E and other oils that are rich in unsaturated fatty acids as well as antioxidants. I have seen the amazing results of such a regimen on friends of mine who followed my advice and achieved motherhood without a single trace of the nine-month stretching period. Vitamin E and other antioxidants carry oxygen to the skin cells and keep the skin pliant and elastic so that the fatty tissue breakdown that causes stretch marks is less likely to occur. In fact, after nine months of this nourishing skin treatment, your skin may well be as soft as your brand-new baby's!

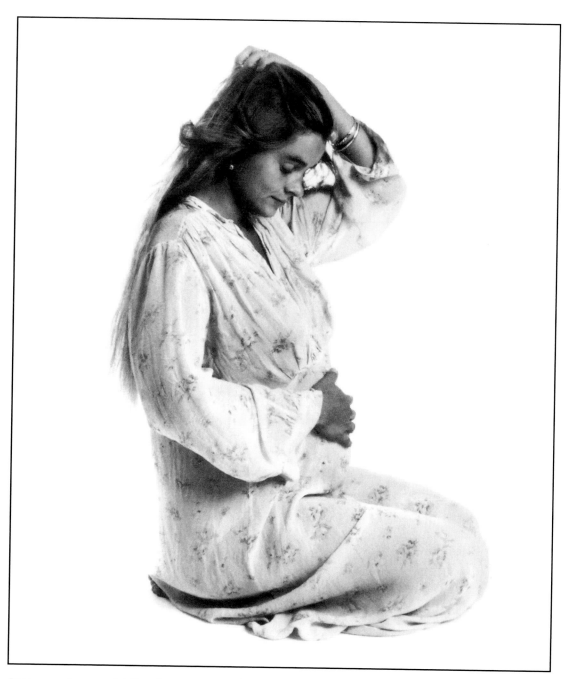

Pregnancy is a special time in a woman's life,
and it calls for special body care.

"Cellulite is a stubborn, mysterious problem. We do know it is not the same as ordinary fat; it can affect you no matter how thin you are."

Another method used for cellulite reduction and body care is the European spa-inspired body wrap. This involves putting on a sauna suit or plastic wrap, then placing blankets over the wrap. Even if it did nothing else for you, the experience of having a body wrap feels so good that it is worth the price of admission. Different spas combine different methods of utilizing various cellulite-fighting ingredients. They are always applied to the body before the body is wrapped or before a sauna suit is put on. One type of wrap utilizes seaweed gel and aloe vera along with essential oils. Another type combines seaweed with mud. Experts in this field of body care say that these wraps help to speed up the elimination of cellulite. Sometimes the plastic wrap is covered with Ace bandages instead of blankets. This procedure keeps the body warm. You then lie down and relax for half an hour to forty-five minutes. After the body wrap is removed, it is followed by a thorough body massage. Following all of this glorious pampering, you are usually led to a stimulating hydro-massage or thalassotherapy-type shower or a seaweed bath soak.

Bathing, of course, is not only therapeutic, relaxing, and stress-reducing, but it is also something you can do in your own home. There are many seaweed bath, shower, and body products on the market today, and even if your budget cannot stretch to include the ticket to a spa for thalassotherapy, you can probably afford to utilize seaweed products in your own home. You can even create your own salt bath by putting three or four cups of coarse kitchen salt or, preferably, sea salt into a tubful of hot water. This makes for the most purifying of baths.

Another method used to fight cellulite is a medically supervised technique from Europe that has the long name of *cellulolipolisis*. This is a form of electric acupuncture and is administered only by physicians. With this technique, long, thin electrodes are inserted superficially into the skin in the targeted areas. The sensation it creates is said to feel like an intense tickling. The process supposedly releases trapped water and fat by stimulating circulation and speeding up fat metabolism. This electrotherapy is combined with a strict low-calorie diet and requires six weekly hour-long visits. It is being used in Europe by at least 1,000 dermatologists and plastic surgeons at this time. A German plastic surgeon, Dr. A. Riedel, says that "if the patient continues dieting, the problematic body parts will never again bulge."[2]

As a last resort for cellulite—and I don't mean a spa in Switzerland!—there are many reputable doctors and plastic surgeons who practice the form of cosmetic surgery known as *liposuction*. If you decide to look into this option, however, please make sure to do proper research with a professional in this area before taking this type of action.

Finally, when fighting cellulite, you must be concerned about what goes into your body. I am not a nutritionist and do not pretend to be one. However, there are certain basic principles that are universally agreed upon by people in the field of nutrition. For instance, a diet high in salt and animal products, particularly those that come from animals raised with the use of hormones, contributes to cellulite. On the other hand, a diet low in fat and high in vitamins A, C, and E, the B vitamins, and minerals helps to fight cellulite. Drinking lots and lots of water improves the metabolism and helps flush out the lymphatic system. A diet that includes plenty of whole grains, vegetables, fruits, and "live foods"—foods that have not been overrefined, overcooked, or overpreserved—helps to correct imbalances in the body. Instead of a diet high in fatty foods and refined carbohydrates, switch to eating whole grains, high-fiber foods, and fruits like pineapples, papayas, melons, and any kind of berries. These foods are very cleansing and detoxifying to the body as a whole.

As I have said throughout this book, science is constantly making new breakthroughs. You may have already heard about aminophylline, an asthma drug that was recently discovered to reduce fat deposits when applied as a cream on the thighs and other fatty areas. The information in the first news report on this development was that

Table 8.1 Step-By-Step Body Care Techniques and Products

This table outlines, step by step, the procedures and products for your basic routine for body skin care, including cellulite control. Use it as a quick reference to the correct types of skin care products, as well as the proper sequence and frequency for using them, for your particular skin type. If you are unsure about what type of skin you have, see Know Your Skin Type on page 34.

SKIN TYPE	FIRST STEP	SECOND STEP	THIRD STEP	FOURTH STEP
	MASSAGE & CELLULITE CONTROL	EPIDERMABRADING & CELLULITE CONTROL	CLEANSING & CELLULITE CONTROL	MOISTURIZING & CELLULITE CONTROL
Normal and Combination Skin	Massage formula/ cellulite treatment, massaged in upward and circular motion (every day).	Body scrub/cellulite treatment, scrubbed vigorously with an upward and circular motion (every day).	pH-balanced body wash or shower and bath gel, followed by towel massage (every day).	Nourishing and moisturizing body lotion, cream, or light oil (every day).
Dry, Very Dry, and Aging Skin	Massage formula/ cellulite treatment, massaged in upward and circular motion (every day).	Body scrub/cellulite treatment, scrubbed vigorously with an upward and circular motion (every day).	pH-balanced body wash or shower and bath gel, followed by towel massage (every day).	Nourishing and moisturizing body lotion, cream, or light oil (every day).
Oily or Acne-Prone Skin	Massage formula/ cellulite treatment, massaged in upward and circular motion (every day).	Body scrub/cellulite treatment, scrubbed vigorously with an upward and circular motion (twice a day on chest and back).	pH-balanced body wash or shower and bath gel, followed by towel massage (every day).	Nourishing and moisturizing body lotion, cream, or light oil (every day).
Sensitive Skin	Massage formula/ cellulite treatment, massaged in upward and circular motion (every day).	Body scrub/cellulite treatment, diluted with water, scrubbed vigorously with an upward and circular motion (every other day).	pH-balanced body wash or shower and bath gel, followed by towel massage (every day).	Nourishing and moisturizing body lotion, cream, or light oil (every day).

aminophylline appeared to speed up the metabolism of fat cells in those specific areas, thereby shrinking the excess fat. George Bray, M.D., of the Pennington Biomedical Research Center at Louisiana State University in Baton Rouge, and Frank Greenway, M.D., an endocrinologist and clinical professor of internal medicine at Harbor UCLA Medical Center in Torrance, California, released the findings of a study conducted on two groups of several women over a five-week period. The results showed a significant improvement, specifically the loss of between 1 and 1.5 inches around the thighs.[3]

As I have noted, the most publicized name for the substance that makes up this brand-new product is aminophylline. However, as it turns out, aminophylline is just one of a whole group of substances called *methylxanthines*. One methylxanthine, called theobromine, is a diuretic that is found in cocoa extract, black tea, green tea, and Paraguay tea. Another methylxanthine is caffeine, which can be derived from coffee beans and also black teas. Because my orientation is toward natural ingredients, I was happy to find out that methylxanthines are present in these natural substances and can do the same job without causing the side effects of the drug aminophylline.

Other high-tech research and development laboratories are putting together formulas with alternative ingredients, and new discoveries and inventions become available all the time. Scientists now say that methylxanthines block the receptors of fat-storing hormones, causing the cells to release, instead of to retain, their fat content.

Dr. Brian Keller of BioZone Labs says, "The difference between alpha-hydroxy acids and the active ingredients in thigh-slimming products is that in the fat reduction products, these ingredients, called methylxanthines, work by decreasing fat deposits below the skin surface. Hydroxy acids, on the other hand, help accelerate skin turnover and improve surface skin appearance, and can get rid of fine lines and wrinkles. The firming and tightening abilities of acids like glycolic, lactic, malic, citric, tartaric, salicylic, and pyruvic have a dramatic effect on the outer layers of skin by helping rebuild the network of collagen and elastin in the lower layers. These support fibers are the foundation of the skin, and when increased by topical application of alpha-hydroxy acids, they can firm and tighten skin tissue."[4] What this means is that, in most cases, the fat-reduction products and the alpha-hydroxy acid products can be used simultaneously, when the desired result is to obtain a slimming effect plus a greater look of elasticity in the skin.

Even with all of the current excitement and hullabaloo over this new fat-reducing wonder cream, I still feel that there is no substitute for a regular program of exercise and epidermabrasion (combined with other special treatments from time to time). This lifelong regimen is absolutely necessary, and it is still the most effective, enjoyable way to treat and pamper your body into looking its most beautiful, sensual, and healthy.

It takes some discipline to care for your body, and especially to reverse unwanted—sometimes genetically determined—tendencies in your body. But I can tell you that whatever work you do will be reflected in your looks, your energy, and the new lust for life that you will feel!

CHAPTER 9

Growing a Great Head of Hair

So far I have been discussing and elaborating on the benefits of epidermabrasion for the facial and body skin. Now I would like to talk about the importance of epidermabrading the scalp and the direct effect this has toward growing a healthy head of hair, while eliminating abnormal hair loss and hair thinning.

There have been many scientific breakthroughs and much controversy over the years regarding hair growth—and its opposite, hair loss, which was once thought of as being strictly hereditary. I am not saying that heredity does not affect hair loss, but more and more ways are being found to counteract this particular condition. We now know that poor circulation, stress, and nutritional deficiencies can contribute to the problem, so correcting these conditions is part of the solution.

IT ALL STARTS WITH A CLEAN, HEALTHY SCALP

As I have discussed, the shedding of dead skin cells goes on all over the body, and this most definitely includes the scalp. The accumulation of dead skin cells on the scalp can clog the ducts of the sebaceous (oil-secreting) glands, leading to embedded deposits of sebum, decreased ventilation and oxygenation, a general weakening of the hair structure, and hair loss. Dandruff may develop as dead cells clump together, becoming large, visible flakes and attracting dust and bacteria. Dandruff too can obstruct normal hair growth.

Stimulating and massaging the scalp help to lift away the dead skin cells and scaly waste matter. They also encourage circulation to the scalp, bringing fresh blood to the roots of the hair. This is vital for cell renewal in the epidermis (the outer skin surface).

Washing the hair frequently—every day or every other day—is the first important step to adhere to. I can already hear some of you with dry hair saying, "But that will make my hair even drier!" Quite the reverse. The increase in circulation you will be creating with a good shampoo/massage will stimulate the oil glands to work more efficiently, thereby helping to bring the natural oils to the hair shaft. If the ends of your hair are damaged or dried out, there are any number of wonderful conditioning shampoos, rinses, and hair packs made with natural proteins, vitamins, and herbal or botanical extracts that can be used to renew and give body to the hair itself. Always make sure to use a shampoo that is pH-balanced.

Using hair conditioners, however, is not a substitute for working on the real basis of hair beauty, which is a super-healthy scalp. So don't worry: Washing the hair frequently will not dry out your hair, unless you use an extremely harsh, alkaline shampoo. Conversely, if you have oily hair, frequent shampooing/massaging will not make your hair oilier, as some people believe. Even though you will be stimulating the oil glands, you will also be keeping your scalp squeaky clean, free of scaly-oily waste material, and unclogging choked hair follicles. A good old-fashioned vinegar rinse can help control excess oil, and will also balance the pH of your scalp and hair. Remember

Grandma's vinegar hair rinse? (Phew! What a smell!) She may not have known it, but she was actually giving you an acidic rinse, in a formula passed down from her ancestors, that helped to make the hair healthy and shiny. Hair and skin science now call this restoring the pH balance. As I've said, our ancestors knew these things, but without the fancy scientific names that we give them today!

By now I imagine you're getting the message that the keys to regenerating the scalp and growing healthy hair are cleansing, stimulation, and epidermabrasion/massage. No matter how good your nutrition is, the nutrients you consume cannot be carried to the scalp if there is poor circulation, resulting in constricted blood vessels. I believe that a pre-shampoo massage, utilizing a mixture of a few very effective natural ingredients, is the key to solving 90 percent of scalp problems and increasing hair growth. My favorite massage formula consists of a combination of two plant extracts, one of which is jojoba oil. According to research conducted by Dr. Javier Gomez, jojoba oil removes embedded sebum deposits from around the hair follicles, cleaning and unclogging them and affording relief from dandruff. This frees the scalp to promote renewed hair growth. Also excellent for the scalp are a number of essential oils, namely rosemary, eucalyptus, henna, cedarwood, juniper, lavender, burdock root, nettle, sage, mint, lemongrass, and thyme (more about essential oils in Chapter 10), as well as herbs like henna, birch, horsetail, yarrow, and hops. I also like capsicum (also known as cayenne or red pepper). All of these herbs and essential oils are known not only for stimulating and conditioning the scalp, but for their antiseptic qualities as well. These ingredients can be found in better health food stores, skin care boutiques, and herb shops. Other ingredients to look for in hair care products include biotin, panthenol (sometimes called d-panthenol or pro-vitamin B_5), and polysorbate-80, all of which are known to benefit both the scalp and the hair.

"Grandma's simple, old-fashioned vinegar rinse is still a good treatment for hair. It restores the proper pH balance of the hair and scalp."

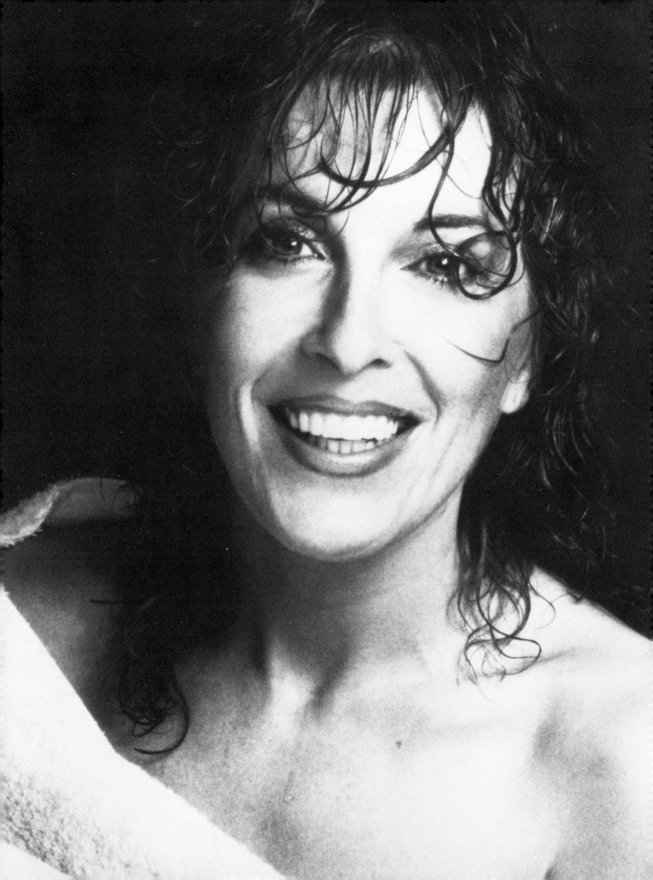

SCALP MASSAGE AND CONDITIONING

I have been asked by so many people—mainly men—what can be done to help fight hair loss or improve the condition of the scalp that I finally developed my own scalp massage formula. After doing the basic research, and realizing how similar this problem was to the problem of regenerating the skin everywhere else on the body, I decided that the best formula would be one that could remove embedded sebum and reactivate hair follicles, and I developed a formula that combines jojoba oil with some specially selected essential oils. I mix this product in my very own home as a gift for friends. You can do the same.

To make your own basic formula, pour two ounces of pure jojoba oil into an empty bottle or jar and add essential oils. You can choose your own combination of essential oils from those mentioned on page 101, but my preference and suggestion is the following: thirty-six drops (approximately one-quarter teaspoon) of peppermint oil; twenty-four drops each of eucalyptus oil, rosemary oil, and lemongrass oil; twelve drops of cedarwood oil; and one-eighth teaspoon of cayenne pepper (powdered capsicum). Blend the essential oils and the capsicum well into the jojoba oil. The aroma of this homemade scalp treatment is quite pungent, but don't let it scare you; the aroma will disappear from your scalp and hair after a thorough shampooing.

The Fingertip Massage

Once you have mixed my scalp massage oil, apply an even amount all over your scalp, enough to moisten your entire scalp. Now, using your fingertips, start massaging vigorously, in the same manner that you would shampoo your hair. Keep applying more of the mixture until your scalp is saturated, and continue to massage for three to five minutes. For best results, do this while bending forward from the waist, with your head hanging down, to allow for extra blood circulation to the scalp. As you massage the mixture into your scalp, you are loosening up accumulated dandruff and getting rid of dead cells and debris. And remember, going back to my original message: Anytime you get rid of dead skin cells (whether on the face, the body, or the scalp), you are encouraging healthy new cells to rise to the surface. Basically, you are epidermabrading your scalp. You are stimulating circulation, allowing the bloodstream to bring needed nutrients to the scalp, and of course you are allowing your scalp to breathe. A scalp that lacks oxygen grows little hair. Many people do not know this and have suffered from both scalp problems and hair loss because of a scalp that was constricted.

After you have massaged your scalp for about five minutes, comb or brush the massage formula through your hair, relax, and leave the mixture on your scalp and hair for another ten to twenty minutes. This will give the hair as well as the scalp a good conditioning treatment. Then shampoo your hair thoroughly with a good pH-balanced shampoo. You may need to lather up two or three times to get out the extra oil, because you've just given your hair a real essential oil treatment. Once your hair is clean, you can finish up with a good pH-balanced finishing rinse if you wish (although chances are you probably won't need one).

I have heard from a number of people who have made and used my scalp massage recipe that the results are well worth the effort. In fact, I have had comments from several men who said that areas where their hair had seemed to be thinning out were looking healthier and fuller. Some have told me that the rate of hair loss decreased considerably; some have said that it stopped completely. How often you will want to give yourself this pre-shampoo massage treatment depends on your particular scalp or hair condition. If you are prone to dandruff and/or thinning hair or balding, or if you simply want to increase your hair growth, you can do it every day. If your scalp and hair are already in good condition, doing it two to three times a week can promote an even healthier, more luxurious mane.

Brushing

You should also massage your scalp by brushing. This can be done after the fingertip massage, while the massage mixture is still on your scalp, or by itself. Brushing distributes the natural oils throughout the hair, removes accumulations of dust and pollutants, stimulates circulation, and gives a sheen to the hair. Brushing too should be done while bending forward from the waist, with your head hanging down. Brush from back to front, giving your scalp at least 50 to 100 brush strokes. Some scalp specialists believe in using a natural bristle brush; others feel that this type of brush, with its tightly packed bristles, can pull at your hair and damage it. I use a Denman brush that has nylon bristles with rounded ends set in a rubber pad. The bristles are set wide apart, so the hair cannot get tangled up in them. This type of brush glides through the hair and gives a great massage. Brushing is best done on either dry or semi-dry hair (such as hair that has the jojoba and essential oil mixture brushed through it). Never brush hair that is soaking wet. Truly wet hair is quite elastic and can be pulled and stretched to the breaking point. Combing with a large, wide-toothed comb is best for wet hair. When combing, it helps to start close to the bottom of the hair and work your way up a little bit at a time. This technique can help you to minimize the amount of hair broken off or pulled out by combing, especially if you have long and/or fine hair.

Daily brushing with a good-quality hairbrush is a must for beatiful hair. I prefer a nylon-bristle brush. To detangle wet hair, use a well-made wide-toothed comb.

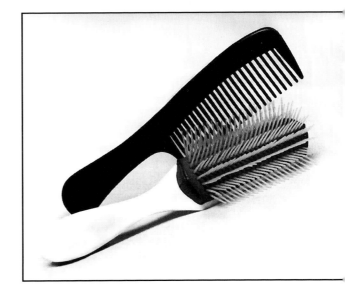

BE KIND TO YOUR HAIR

Finally, there are a number of common-sense precautions you can take that can prevent unnecessary hair loss. For example, there is a condition called *traction alopecia* that is characterized by a receding hairline and that is found in women, children, and some men. This occurs when the hair is pulled too tightly for too long, such as in a ponytail or in a tight chignon like those worn by dancers, athletes, and models. The pressure this puts on the roots of the hair can cause hair loss to occur at the hairline. This condition can be very traumatic. To avoid it, try to keep rubber bands out of your hair; if you must use them, try to keep your hair tied very loosely.

Wearing hats or wigs on a regular basis can also also cause problems, because this can reduce the blood circulation and therefore the supply of oxygen, endangering the scalp. If you do wear hats often, make sure to give yourself some time off, as well as a good vigorous massage in between wearings.

For additional scalp circulation and relaxation, try lying on a slant board with your feet elevated, your head down, and your spine straight for about fifteen minutes a day. This is good for the entire body and really enlivens the complexion. The yoga headstand (a position described in any good yoga book) is also great for sending blood surging through the scalp. If you cannot do that, the somewhat easier neck-stand will do the job of increasing the circulation to the face and scalp. Yoga experts say it also promotes the health of the thyroid gland.

My main concern in this chapter has been with promoting the health of the scalp, which is the basis for healthy hair and hair growth, rather than with hair styling or the treatment of individual hair types. If you refer to Appendix I, A Glossary of Nature's Bountiful Gifts, you will find a list of the proteins, vitamins, herbs, and botanicals, such as panthenol, keratin, henna, biotin, etc., that make for the best shampoos, rinses, conditioning treatments, and hair packs. I advise you to experiment with a variety of hair care preparations that contain these fine natural ingredients in order to find the ones that best suit your particular hair type. The largest selection of these natural products is probably to be found in your local health food store.

I like using suma, babassu, agave, copaiba, awapuhi, and other rain forest botanicals on my hair. The use of these botanicals not only beautifies the hair and scalp, but can also help the people who live in the world's rain forests, as these exotic ingredients are obtained from *sustainably harvested plants.* This term means that the ingredients are obtained without destroying the plants' root foundations, allowing them to flourish and grow for years. Sustainable harvesting of rain forest botanicals promotes the health of the ecosystem, which in turn supports the lives of indigenous people and animals.

Just as with my regimens for face and body care, the elements of desire, time, and energy are involved in caring for your scalp and hair. But if you make the commitment to try it, you will find that the results are well worth the effort.

CHAPTER 10

The Once-a-Week, Super-Easy, At-Home Salon Facial

Now that you are getting the basic daily routine under your belt—and hopefully by now it is becoming automatic—I am going to suggest that you give yourself a once-a-week super facial. It will give you a glorious feeling and make you look terrific. You'll think you have been transported to a European facial salon! My once-a-week facial is a great thing to do before going out for a night on the town, or on a Sunday night before starting a new work week.

STEP ONE: CLEANSING AND STEAMING

First of all, start with your regular cleansing massage. Towel off and go on to your scrub-massage, doing each step with the exercise positions as described in Chapter 2. While the scrub is still on your face, give yourself a five-minute facial steaming. You can do this with a small facial sauna machine (available at many department stores and drugstores) or simply—and less expensively—with a pot of boiling water

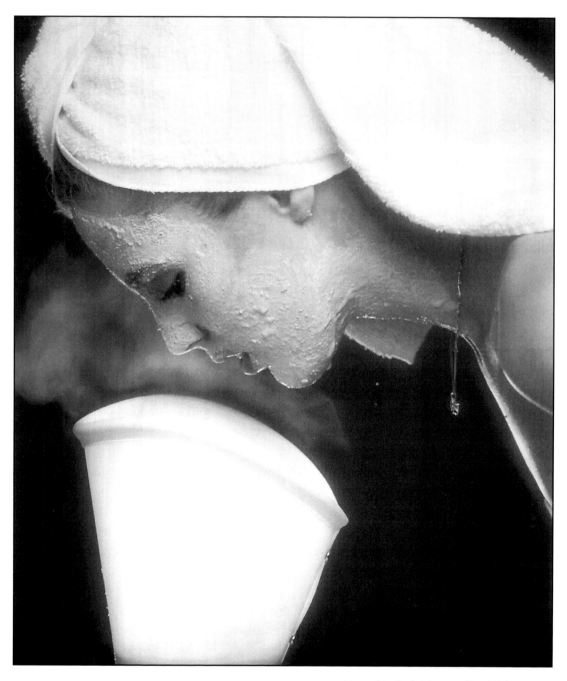

A weekly facial is an affordable luxury
you won't want to do without!

and a towel. Boil a pot of water on the stove (any ordinary pot will do) and put the pot on top of a trivet or thick potholder on a table.

If you wish, you can add several drops of your favorite essential oil or oils to the water. Sit in a comfortable position and lean your face over the pot of water. Then, with a big bath towel, make a "tent" covering both your head and the pot, so that the steam rises up to your face. (Be sure to keep your face a comfortable distance from the pot—you don't want to burn or irritate your skin.) Stay in this position for about five minutes. This will open the pores and allow the scrub (and any essential oils you use) to penetrate and cleanse more deeply. It will also stimulate circulation and leave your skin rosy and radiant, as well as opening your nasal passages so that you will be able to breathe more freely. After five minutes, wash the scrub off your face with warm water and gently towel dry.

STEP TWO: THE CLAY-BASED MASK

You are ready for the next step, the clay-based mask. Apply the mask all over your face and neck (and, if you wish, on certain areas of your body) and lie down for a good twenty-minute rest and relaxation period. If you like, put on some mellow music to help create a happy state of mind. After the twenty minutes are up, wash off the mask with warm water, towel dry, and apply your skin toner or astringent and let it dry naturally.

STEP THREE: MOISTURIZING AND NOURISHING

You are now ready for your last step, which is the moisturizing and nourishing massage. Apply your firming gel primer, followed by a good moisturizer or nourishing cream, repeating, once again, your exercise positions and massage techniques. If you are doing the facial before going to bed, use your regular nighttime nourishing treatment. If you are going out, use a moisturizer or very light textured, not-too-oily nourishing cream for the massage—you do not want your face to appear too shiny.

AND NOW . . . THE TRUTH ABOUT MAKEUP

At this point you may be asking, "What about makeup? Dare I apply makeup to this beautifully cleansed skin?" The answer may surprise you.

After many years of assisting women with their skin care problems and answering numerous questions on the subject, I have discovered an interesting phenomenon: Most women have been taught to believe that makeup is bad for their skin. I am now going to take a firm stand on this subject—and surprise you, if you are one of the many women who has been living with this misconception. *Makeup is good for your skin.* In fact, not only can makeup benefit your skin, but it is one of the greatest tools available to aid in slowing and even reversing the aging process of the face.

Why? It is a simple matter of protection versus exposure. It becomes more and more obvious, especially as the years go by, that body skin tends to retain its smooth texture and youthful appearance, while facial skin develops lines and dryness much more rapidly. An obviously weather-beaten, aging appearance develops.

If you haven't already guessed what I'm leading up to, it's quite simple. Our body skin is clothed at least 90 percent of the time. This of course makes it difficult for the sun's ultraviolet rays to do damage and have an aging effect on the skin. Our facial skin, on the other hand, is exposed most of the time, so it is the most vulnerable part of all.

Most people don't realize that they needn't lie out in the sun to do damage to their skin. Dermatologists and skin scientists have proved that exposure to UVA and UVB rays takes place every day as you walk down the street.

But take heart, and don't worry. You don't have to hide in your house or wear a veil. Every problem has a solution. This is where a good moisturizer and good makeup foundation come in.

A good moisturizer that contains a sunscreen should be applied underneath your foundation, or makeup base. This will ensure the utmost supply of moisture to the skin. When makeup foundation is applied over the moisturizer, together they create a protective barrier against the external elements.

CHOOSING MAKEUP PRODUCTS

There are many different types of foundation on the market. All makeup foundations contain an ingredient called titanium dioxide. This is the same substance that is the latest in natural sunscreen technology (see page 81), and that is found in that white ointment you often see on lifeguards' noses. Titanium dioxide has always been present in all makeup foundation, and it gives great protection against all external elements. (No wonder women who wore makeup all their lives ended up with younger looking skin than their friends who didn't!) Today, titanium dioxide is micronized—reduced to powder particles tiny enough to be invisible. My favorite type of product is a liquid foundation that gives good coverage—meaning that it minimizes any imperfections—while giving a totally natural, unmade-up look to the skin.

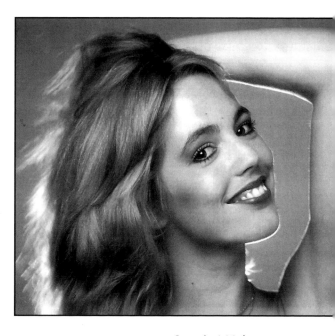

Surprise! Makeup is good for your skin.

I have devoted my career to formulating products utilizing natural ingredients, so it was natural that I would endeavor to develop a makeup foundation with a natural oil base and nutrient ingredients. After experimenting with several different vegetable oils, I found I achieved the best results with jojoba oil. This oil is derived from the jojoba seed, and has proven to be highly effective in rejuvenating and improving the health of both the scalp and the hair. After extensive lab research, it was found to give equal benefits when used in skin care products—that is, it has a smoothing, regenerating effect on the skin. When I used jojoba oil in my makeup foundation, I found to my delight that it worked equally well on oily, normal, and dry skin types. In other words, it was neither too greasy nor too drying.

I have applied this same concept of using natural nutrient ingredients in all my other makeup products, from lipsticks to eye shadows to blushes, with great success. I therefore know with certainty that makeup formulated with these natural ingredients is not only beneficial to your skin, but can also make you look gorgeous.

I am happy to say that the philosophy I have always espoused is spreading throughout the makeup industry. This is the idea that makeup can also be a treatment product. Aside from the protective factors, you will now find that moisturizing and anti-wrinkle complexes, oil-control formulas, and many other ingredients and technologies that are used in the new and advanced skin care products are increasingly being incorporated into makeup as well. The inclusion of ingredients beneficial to specific skin problems provides for a continuum of treatment.

Just be sure when you buy makeup that the product contains a preservative system to keep it from going rancid. If you are going to buy a lipstick with natural ingredients, it is a good idea to smell it before you buy it. If it smells rancid, do not buy it. Always remember that rancidity causes free-radical formation, and the lack of correct preservatives can cause serious bacterial infections.

Now that you know what good makeup can do for your skin, it behooves you to research and explore the natural cosmetic market and try different products to see which ones appeal to your particular taste and suit your needs the best. Remember, the right makeup will not only make you look and feel beautiful, but it will also greatly aid in reversing the aging process of your face for years to come.

CHAPTER 11

My Unique Approach to Aromatherapy and Color Therapy in Skin Care

I have always been devoted to exploring and utilizing the benefits with which we are so wonderfully endowed in all our five senses: smell, sight, touch, taste, and hearing. My career in music—in the form of singing, writing songs, and playing the piano—encompasses the world of sound. The other four senses are reflected and utilized in my work with natural skin care, body care, and make-up products. I want to focus now on the senses of smell and sight—as manifested in aromatherapy and color therapy—and how I have applied these two arts/sciences to my skin care philosophy.

During the time I spent studying and doing extensive research on skin care and physiology, I included in my work the subjects of aromatherapy, color therapy, and various techniques of healing with scents and colors. The further I delved into the subject, the more interested and excited I became. I found that the very instincts we have as young children—being attracted to and playing with smells and colors—are not just basic human tendencies, but are also manifestations of inner intuitive powers that have the ability to heal our bodies and minds all the rest of our lives. As is true in so many other ways, we have much to learn from children and their instinctive responses to life and nature.

THE POWER OF AROMA AND COLOR

"Has a particular smell ever transported you to another place and time, bringing back memories you hadn't even been aware of a moment earlier? This common experience shows the mysterious power of fragrance."

The arts of aromatherapy and color therapy have been used since ancient times (here we go again!), but now they are backed up by modern scientific research. Research has been done proving the benefits of using aroma and color to treat all kinds of problems, both psychological and physiological. Scientific studies tell us how olfactory (smell) and visual (color) messages reinforce each other as they are sent to the brain. When used together, messages sent by aroma and color therapy work to unite the senses, allowing the brain to receive much stronger impressions then when they are used separately.

When we perceive a certain smell or color, a response is triggered in the psyche on an unconscious level. This in turn effects a physiological response. Smell and color are perceived and responded to simultaneously on the mental, physical, and spiritual planes. Almost all of us have had the dramatic experience of smelling something that suddenly brings back a time, place, or event in our lives that we might not have remembered at all if not for this unconscious association. With some simple education and knowledge, you can use this amazing power of association consciously, by choosing which responses are most beneficial for you, as an individual, to create in yourself.

According to Eastern philosophy, our bodies have seven energy centers also referred to as *chakras*. These centers channel energy to the various organs of the body to keep the body and mind working in perfect balance. Each center is governed by a specific color ray. This can even be seen, through the use of Kirlian photography. This is a photographic technique that can be used to capture an image of an electromagnetic field; in the case of a human being, we would say that it results in a picture of an individual's aura. When we meditate

on or visualize a specific color, it has a strong stimulating and healing impact on the particular chakra, or energy center, associated with
it. The same principle applies to aromas. Each and every smell has
its own specific effect on one or more chakra or energy center. The
vibration of each aroma or color is a form of energy, and this energy
activates a particular center in the body.

Aromatherapy has really been used for thousands of years, in the
form of the burning of incense. The ancient Egyptians burned aromatic substances to please their gods; in many ancient cultures, it
was believed that certain aromas would get rid of evil spirits. There
was once a legend (still popular among some people) that said if you
placed rosemary under your pillow while you slept, it would dispel
nightmares. Incense has been used in all kinds of religions and hous-
es of worship to bring about a calm and meditative state. It comes in
many scents that have calming effects, including rose, jasmine, san-
dalwood, oriental spices, and others. The Japanese have been experimenting with, using, and documenting the effectiveness of mint and
citrus essences for the purpose of inducing alertness. This practice is
also now being used in many other countries. When placed in such a
way that they permeate offices and other work environments, these
scents have been proven to increase productivity. Similar examples
can be found of the use of color therapy. Rooms in many hospitals,
health spas, and salons are now painted soft, soothing shades of
aqua, blue, and lavender. Yellow and yellow-orange, on the other
hand, are used in workplaces to increase energy, alertness, and effi-
ciency. Children's schools and nurseries have to be painted vibrant
and beautiful colors, or the children don't even want to stay or play
in them. Children are smart. They don't want to feel sad or de-
pressed. Dr. Bernard Jensen, a well-known proponent of natural
healing, has said, "Color is a food. It feeds the body, soul, and mind.
I find people are starving for color and a lot of them don't even know
it. I believe that our bodies will repair and rebuild in the presence of
beautiful colors. It's absolutely a necessity."

APPLICATIONS OF AROMATHERAPY AND COLOR THERAPY

"You can even coordinate the color of the clothes you are wearing with the scent you splash on. What fun!"

Now that you understand something of how aroma and color therapy work, let me explain how I have always applied these principles to my skin care products. After spending several years doing research and experimentation to determine which herbs, vitamins, and other natural substances bring about the greatest results in treating the skin—which after all is the largest organ of the body—I realized that truly complete treatment should also incorporate the correct aromatic and color vibrations. I use specific essences or smells to reinforce the visual message of colors being sent to the brain, and vice versa. The use of aromatherapy with color therapy works toward uniting the senses to receive a strong impression, both olfactorily and visually. In each of my products, the aroma and color key reemphasize the function and purpose of the particular product. For example, in my moisturizers and in my Rainforest line of products, I use essences derived from nature's bountiful supply of moisture-full green botanicals and plants. These essences are accompanied by the color key of green. The green scent combined with the green color key sends to the brain a sensory message of nature's harmony, balance, and moisture renewal. The benefit of this is not only healthy skin, but a feeling of total health and well-being of mind and body as well. Another example is my French Massage Formula, which includes a complex of botanicals that has the double purpose of improving circulation and also inducing relaxation. The essence combines the soft, languid, and romantic florals of jasmine and gardenia with an accent of mood-elevating carnation. The color keys are quieting pastels like aqua and lavender to violet, which have been used for thousands of years to induce a meditative state of well-being.

Table 11.1 offers a synopsis of how aroma and color coordinate in a magical synergy. These are just a few of the many qualities in the interactions between color and fragrance—there are many more.

Table 11.1 Coordinating Color Therapy and Aromatherapy

The table below shows how color and aroma are coordinated with each other. Notice how similar the effects of the various color rays are to the effects of the aromas associated with them.

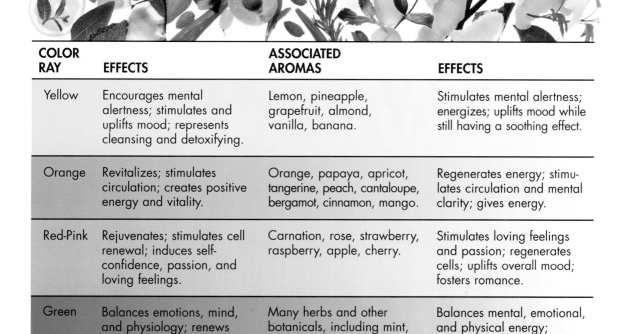

COLOR RAY	EFFECTS	ASSOCIATED AROMAS	EFFECTS
Yellow	Encourages mental alertness; stimulates and uplifts mood; represents cleansing and detoxifying.	Lemon, pineapple, grapefruit, almond, vanilla, banana.	Stimulates mental alertness; energizes; uplifts mood while still having a soothing effect.
Orange	Revitalizes; stimulates circulation; creates positive energy and vitality.	Orange, papaya, apricot, tangerine, peach, cantaloupe, bergamot, cinnamon, mango.	Regenerates energy; stimulates circulation and mental clarity; gives energy.
Red-Pink	Rejuvenates; stimulates cell renewal; induces self-confidence, passion, and loving feelings.	Carnation, rose, strawberry, raspberry, apple, cherry.	Stimulates loving feelings and passion; regenerates cells; uplifts overall mood; fosters romance.
Green	Balances emotions, mind, and physiology; renews strength physically and mentally; creates harmony; helps soothe nerves.	Many herbs and other botanicals, including mint, lime, cucumber, vetiver, melon, pear, guava, kiwi, sea algae.	Balances mental, emotional, and physical energy; refreshes, renews; helps soothe and stabilize nerves.
Blue-Turquoise	Cools, soothes; helps mental focus and concentration; relaxes.	Blueberry, juniper berries, cassis, blue violet, chamomile, blue sea algae.	Cools, soothes, relaxes, reduces stress.
Purple-Violet-Lavender	Calms; promotes peacefulness; relaxes; reduces stress; soothes; tranquilizes; enhances meditation.	Violet, lilac, jasmine, grape, hyacinth, wisteria, purple berries.	Soothes and tranquilizes; promotes romance, sensuality.

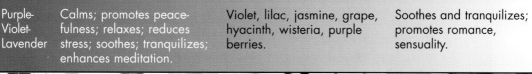

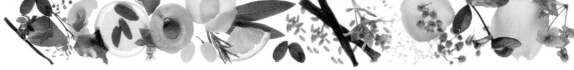

The Intrigue of Fragrance

Color and aroma have the power to stimulate the mind and the senses, further accentuating the benefits of any particular treatment. This is why I always incorporate the elements of color and scent when formulating my products.

Where I completely veer off and disagree with the aromatherapy "purists" is that I extend my field of aromatherapy much further than they do. They use only *volatile essential oils*. An essential oil is a basically pure and extremely pungent extract from an herb or other plant that is used for therapeutic and medicinal purposes. It is never used in its concentrated form in the same way as a fragrance or perfume is. I certainly do utilize essential oils and agree with the basic premises of their uses and actions. But what most people do not know is that all fragrances have, within their very bases, combinations of different pure essential oils. For example, when chemists or perfumers make up fragrances, they always start out with a pure essential oil or oils and then use special enhancers to give a fragrance the specific notes—very much like the use of musical notes—that they want to achieve. Among perfumers in the perfume industry, fragrances are described as combinations of bottom notes, middle notes, and top notes. I find it absolutely fascinating. Unbelievable as it may seem, a banana fragrance contains a blend of pure essential orange oil, spearmint oil, and pettigrain oil. A carnation fragrance starts out with a base of clove

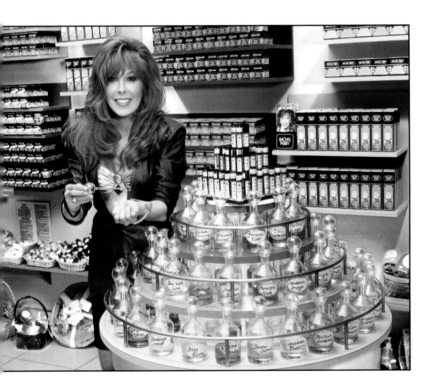

oil, bay leaf oil, cedarwood oil, amyris oil, bois de rose oil, and gal-banum oil, all of which are all pure essential oils. The fragrance of lilac starts out with a base of pure ylang-ylang and orange essential oils. The mystique of fragrance chemistry has been evolving for centuries and continues to reach higher dimensions through modern technology. The things that can be achieved by a perfumer are an absolutely amazing combination of art and science. Each of the world's most brilliant, artistic, and scientific perfumers is quite appropriately called a "nose."

Having been in the health food and natural cosmetics industry for many years, I have observed that people in general have been led to believe that everything that is all natural is good, and anything that contains man-made or synthesized materials is bad. This is just not true. In fact, it is a misunderstanding and distortion of reality. For example, at one time there was a company that sold a makeup product that came from the earth and was entirely natural. It was, however, completely unrefined, and it caused so many allergic skin reactions that it had to be taken off the market. There are lipsticks available that are supposedly all natural, with no preservatives in them. Because of this, there is danger not only of contamination but also of rancidity, which causes the development of free radicals. This is far more dangerous than the use of a preservative made out of a synthetic material. Without effective synthetic and biochemical preservative systems, cosmetics and skin care products are vulnerable to bacterial contamination that can lead to diseases as virulent as pseudomonas infections of the eyes, which can cause blindness. Other fungal or bacterial skin infections can also result if the proper use of preservatives in skin care and makeup products is not adhered to. Yet consumers are misled into believing that everything *completely natural* is totally benevolent and beneficial.

My philosophy has always been to use as many natural ingredients in place of synthetics as I can, but not to rule out modern biochemistry in matters affecting the safety and the improvement of each product. This concept applies also to the creation of fragrance. Even though a fragrance may start out with pure essential oils, the final result is a combination of many, many different elements, both natural and man-made, compounded in a very highly sophisticated and scientific art form. Before I was in the actual business of formulating skin care products, I, too, innocently thought that strawberry-scented cream was made with only fresh strawberries from the garden. When I found out that this was not so, I was, at first, quite disillusioned. However, I then learned that combining nature and science could offer wonderful solutions without compromising either nature or safety.

I believe that all essences and flavors—from fruits, florals, and spices to flavors like vanilla, almond, and so on—have a vital effect on a person's psychological and physiological state. In fact, that is why the fragrance industry has historically had such an impact on society and the art of perfumery has been so highly respected as creative, fascinating, and alluring, as well as being mystical and romantic, for hundreds and hundreds of years. As unbelievable as it may sound, there are 40 million chemically sensitive aroma receptors in the nose, and the power of scent goes straight from our noses to our brains and affects our entire physiology.

Another interesting development related to our sense of smell involves a special type of chemical, called a pheromone, that is secreted through the skin cells of all animals, including humans. In recent years, there has been an increase in the amount of scientific investigation into, and tantalizing evidence of, what these pheromones are all about, and it is proving to be very exciting. Dr. David Moran of the University of Pennsylvania states that there is certain evidence that pheromones are involved in a kind of unconscious communication on a level that goes beyond all the five senses. Many scientists are now calling it a sixth sense. This is due to the fact that although this process involves the olfactory nerve, which is normally involved in the sense of smell, pheromones actually have no perceptible scent. They are odorless natural substances that are released into the air, become airborne, and are received by the vomeronasal organ in the nose. This organ had long been neglected by the scientific community, but has recently come to the forefront of research. Pheromones are then transmitted directly to the hypothalamus, a part of the brain that is responsible for regulating body temperature and other aspects of metabolism. Pheromones may thus have the potential to affect the body's processes at their most basic level. Biologist Dr. Winifred Cutler says that the more specific substance of which pheromones are composed is a hormone called DHEA. This hormone is secreted through the sweat glands and promotes not only feelings of well-being but also of sexual attraction. Pheromones are now being duplicated by fragrance biochemists.

"The instincts we have as young children—being attracted to and playing with smells and colors—are manifestations of inner intuitive powers that have the ability to heal our bodies and minds all the rest of our lives."

Smelling Away the Pounds— Aromatherapy and Weight Loss

I am approaching this with a bit of humor. I recently saw a report by a Chicago-based doctor named Alan Hirsch, who is with the Smell and Taste Research Foundation. He has been doing studies with over-weight people on the direct connection between the olfactory bulb (the nerve at the top of the nose) and the area of the brain that gives you the feeling of being satisfied from eating a food that you like. He has his test subjects utilize inhalers filled with various scents. Every time they become hungry, they sniff their favorite scents—chocolate, banana, vanilla, green apple, etc.—three times with each nostril. Dr. Hirsch reported that almost all of his subjects experienced improvement in weight loss.

I was rather fascinated when I heard this because I have been doing something very similar in my product line for many years. In my lip balm, I use natural fragrances and tastes. In fact, I have always called it a non-fattening taste treat. What I never realized was that this form of smell and taste might actually prove to be meaningful in terms of weight loss. The research on this hasn't yet been as extensive as it will be in the future—but what may seem a little far-fetched at the moment could prove to be well within the realm of possibility.

ESSENTIAL OILS

Since you may not have any familiarity with essential oils, I would like to give you some basic information about what they are and how you can use them to experiment with aromatherapy on your own. I must tell you also that there are many, many books on the market completely dedicated to the study of essential oils.

Pure essential oils are highly concentrated distilled essences of plants that are used for medicinal and therapeutic purposes. These oils are considered to be the very life force of flowers, plants, and trees, and are extremely powerful when used therapeutically.

There are over 100 different essential oils available today. These can be purchased at aromatherapy stores, as well as at some better health food shops, herb shops, and cosmetic boutiques. Thirty-two of the essential oils I have found to be most useful are listed in Table 11.2, together with their specific properties. Use this table to help you choose the essential oils you'd like to experiment with. Always remember, essential oils are very concentrated. Many of them smell extremely pungent, medicinal, and volatile, and they are not meant to be used in the same way as a fragrance or perfume. Although fragrances often start out with bases of essential oils, they are always blended with other ingredients to end up in a much more sophisticated and complex orchestration. Also, when you experiment with essential oils, keep in mind that essential oils should never be taken internally, and should never be applied in their undiluted form directly on the skin. They must always be diluted in either oil or water first.

Table 11.2 Essential Oils and Their Properties

This table lists thirty-two of the essential oils I have found to be the most valuable, together with the special properties of each. Use it to help you choose which oil or oils you would like to experiment with. For instructions on different ways you can use essential oils, see page 130.

ESSENTIAL OIL	PROPERTIES
Angelica	Angelica oil has an earthy, peppery aroma. When inhaled, it acts as a decongestant for the respiratory tract. It also helps to calm nerves and soothe digestive disorders, and is used as an overall detoxifier.
Bergamot	Refreshing and uplifting, bergamot oil is used to relieve anxiety, depression, and nervous tension. It is often used in treatments for oily or acne-prone skin because of its antiseptic and astringent qualities.
Bois de rose (rosewood)	Bois de rose oil calms nerves, balances moods, and alleviates depression. It is used in skin care products to soothe and soften dry skin.
Camphor	Camphor oil is used in skin care products as a detoxifier to help clean up blemished or acne-prone skin. It helps to purify the air and eliminate odors when placed around the room; it is also known to strengthen nerves.
Cedarwood	Used for its harmonizing and stabilizing effects and earthy aroma, this oil can enhance a meditative state. It is also used in skin care products as an anti-inflammatory.
Chamomile	A popular component of many skin and body care products designed to soothe and oxygenate the skin, chamomile is also known to calm nervous tension and decrease anxiety and depression.
Cistus	Recommended as a relaxant, this oil has been known as an aphrodisiac. It blends well with other essential oils.
Clary sage	Clary sage oil acts as a relaxant for both emotional and muscular tension, and is also known as an aphrodisiac. This oil is used to clarify, revitalize, and help detoxify all types of skin.
Clove	Widely used to ease pain of toothaches and gum infections due to its antiseptic and analgesic qualities, clove oil is also included in hair products for scalp stimulation. It has an uplifting, festive aroma.

125

ESSENTIAL OIL	PROPERTIES
Cypress	Psychologically uplifting, cypress has an astringent quality when used in products for oily skin. It can be used for a refreshing bath.
Eucalyptus	Eucalyptus oil has been used for centuries as a decongestant for respiratory problems, especially in steam inhalations. It is also widely used in skin care products for its astringent and purifying properties.
Frankincense	Frankincense is used to induce a meditative state and to reduce anxiety and restlessness. It is also used in skin care products to help rejuvenate the skin.
Freesia	Used to refresh the mind and spirit, this sweet, lemony oil is used in many fragrance products for its invigorating properties.
Geranium	Energizing and uplifting geranium is used to alleviate tension, anxiety, and premenstrual discomforts. It is widely used in skin care products to help control oily skin.
Hyssop	Hyssop oil is known for its harmonizing and balancing effects on the mind and body. Hyssop is also used to reduce and ease skin inflammation.
Juniper	Juniper oil is used to promote clarity of mind and both energize and soothe the body. Juniper makes an invigorating addition to the bath and a great detoxifier in skin care products.
Lavender	Lavender is known for its great ability to restore balance—mentally, physically, and emotionally. It has been used for years as a fragrance and in skin care products designed to soothe inflammation.
Melissa	Melissa oil is known to calm and relax the senses and to help with insomnia. It is also a soothing anti-inflammatory for the skin.
Myrrh	Myrrh is used in skin care products for its soothing, smoothing, and cooling effects. When inhaled, myrrh oil can reduce stress.
Neroli	Neroli oil is a very effective stress reducer that uplifts the spirits. It is also used in astringents for its rejuvenating quality.
Patchouli	Patchouli is a woodsy, earthy oil that is used as an aphrodisiac-type fragrance for both women and men.
Peppermint	Peppermint oil can help focus the mind. It is suggested as a cleanser and refresher for the skin, an energizer for the body, and a soother of aching muscles. It is also great for relief of upset stomach.

ESSENTIAL OIL	PROPERTIES
Pine	Like the scent of a walk in the woods, pine oil's fresh and cleansing aroma is used to purify everything from the body to the air around us. It is recommended as an oil for a soothing bath.
Rosemary	The astringent qualities of rosemary oil make it suitable for use in many skin care products for oily skin. When mixed with jojoba oil, it makes a tremendously effective scalp massage for fine or thinning hair.
Sandalwood	Sandalwood oil, with its woodsy, sweet, spicy aroma, is widely used for meditation and as a fragrance for both men and women. It is also known as an aphrodisiac.
Spearmint	A first cousin to peppermint, spearmint oil is also rich in menthol and has similar effects. It is stimulating and invigorating, and when used in bath gels and body lotions, it is the best thing for cooling the body down on a hot day. It is also great when combined with peppermint to soothe aching muscles and help in cellulite reduction.
Tuberose	Tuberose oil has a sensual aroma that acts as a mild aphrodisiac. Perfumers commonly use it to mix and blend with other fragrances because of its enhancing qualities.
Tea tree	Known for its natural antiseptic qualities, tea tree oil can be used to detoxify and alleviate inflammation in many parts of the body.
Vetiver	Vetiver oil has a wonderful citrusy and woodsy aroma that is relaxing and uplifting. It is used in skin care products for its regenerating and enlivening effects.
White ginger	White ginger oil has a delightful aroma that makes a wonderfully refreshing and stimulating addition to bath, body, and skin care products.
Wintergreen	Wintergreen oil is a sweet, refreshing oil that is used for aching muscles and makes for a great foot massage. Wintergreen can be used for facial steaming to invigorate and purify the skin.
Ylang-ylang	Ylang-ylang oil has an exotic aroma with relaxing effects. Known to be an aphrodisiac, this oil is used by many perfumers to enhance other fragrances and make them longer lasting.

Aromatherapy Recipes

Aromatherapy has many uses in health and beauty care. One of the things aromatherapy is excellent for is enhancing one's mental and/or emotional state. Depending on what effect you want to achieve, you can experiment with any of the oils listed in Table 11.2, or you can try one or more of my recipes for special combinations of essential oils.

To use these recipes, blend the suggested oils together in a clean container with an airtight cover. The combined oils can then be diluted in either oil (for use as a massage oil or fragrance) or water (to be used in a spray mister). Or you can add several drops to a bathtub or a bowl of steaming water to make a soothing or reviving bath or inhalation (see page 130 for specific instructions).

• **To boost mental alertness,** try one of the following combinations:

1. 4 drops patchouli; 4 drops rosewood; 2 drops pine.
2. 5 drops peppermint; 5 drops clove.
3. 2 drops peppermint; 3 drops bergamot; 5 drops vetiver.

• **To increase energy**, try one of the following combinations:

1. 3 drops bergamot; 3 drops rosemary; 4 drops freesia.
2. 3 drops eucalyptus; 3 drops peppermint; 2 drops spearmint; 2 drops cypress.

3. 3 drops spearmint; 3 drops peppermint; 4 drops white ginger.

- **For a centering and balancing effect,** try one of the following combinations:

    1. 3 drops lavender; 3 drops bergamot; 3 drops juniper; 2 drops hyssop.
    2. 3 drops myrrh; 3 drops frankincense; 3 drops sandal-wood; 3 drops vetiver; 3 drops cedarwood.

- **To heighten feelings of romance,** try one of the following combinations:

    1. 4 drops ylang-ylang; 2 drops bergamot; 2 drops neroli; 2 drops tuberose.
    2. 2 drops vetiver; 4 drops ylang-ylang; 3 drops bergamot; 2 drops neroli.
    3. 2 drops tuberose; 2 drops ylang-ylang; 2 drops patchouli; 2 drops cistus; 2 drops sandalwood.

- **To aid relaxation,** try one of the following combinations:

    1. 5 drops geranium; 5 drops neroli.
    2. 4 drops patchouli; 6 drops frankincense; 2 drops bergamot.
    3. 3 drops lavender; 4 drops sandalwood; 3 drops melissa.
    4. 5 drops neroli; 5 drops chamomile.
    5. 3 drops lavender; 4 drops clary sage; 3 drops angelica.

The following are some of the ways of using essential oils that you can experiment with:

• **Baths.** An essential oil bath can be just the soothing, uplifting, and therapeutic experience you need after a long day of work—or whenever you need a special indulgence. Aromatherapy bath treatments can relieve skin conditions while also helping to reduce stress and tension. Add ten to twenty drops of your preferred oil, or combination of oils, to a warm bath and mix well. Sink into your therapeutic bath for at least ten to twenty minutes and enjoy the benefits.

• **Massage.** Make an aromatherapy massage oil by blending essential oil with any type of vegetable oil. Personally, I feel twenty-five to forty drops of essential oil in an eight-ounce container of vegetable oil is an average, safe place to start. If you desire a stronger or weaker solution, test it by adding a few drops at a time and testing the solution on your skin as you go along to make sure it is not irritating and that it meets your particular preference. Just be careful; essential oils are volatile and powerful, and you don't want to irritate vulnerable areas of your body, such as the eyes or mucous membranes. Have a happy massage!

• **Inhalations.** Inhalations aid in the treatment of sinus or respiratory congestion, insomnia, and other conditions. For a steam inhalation, add eight to ten drops of an essential oil, or combination of oils, to a sink or large bowl full of steaming water, lean over the water, and drape a towel over your head to capture the steam. Spend at least five to ten minutes under the towel, breathing in the aroma. You can take frequent breaks if the steam gets too hot, but continue for at least ten minutes. Another steam inhalation method is to use an inhalation recipe with an aromatic diffuser or vaporizer to disperse and diffuse vapors throughout the room. You can also drop an essential oil or oils onto a tissue or pillow to be smelled throughout the day or as you are falling asleep.

• **Spray mister.** Add eight to ten drops of your favorite essential oil, or combination of oils, to water in an eight-ounce mister, shake it up, and spray the mixture on yourself and into the air surrounding you for a change in mood and atmosphere.

• **Generate a party atmosphere.** Add five to ten drops of an essential oil such as rosewood, eucalyptus, and/or white ginger to a bowl of warm water to enliven a stale room. Drop about ten drops of an essential oil such as clove, eucalyptus, or cedarwood on a fireplace log before burning it.

I know that with a little experimentation, you'll come to experience the full benefits of essential oils, as I have. I hope that you can experiment and enjoy the sensory joys and benefits to be derived from combining color, smell, and taste with your other senses, and that the introduction I've given you in this chapter will inspire you to look further into these fascinating subjects.

CHAPTER 12

Age Is an Attitude:
Five Decades in the Life
of a Beautiful Woman

I would like to conclude this book with the real-life story of a woman who has been dedicated to the belief and inner knowledge—and is living proof of the fact—that age is an attitude. Her name is Sheryl Carson. Sheryl's attitude is reflected in the continual evolution of her beauty from one decade to the next, as you can see from the photographs I have compiled from five of these decades—fifty years! As you can see, my friend Sheryl was, is, and always will be a beautiful woman. She has had a great influence on my life, and has made me to want to convey her wisdom to other women who may need to understand the enduring power of their own femininity and how their own mindset influences the way they look and how they are perceived by others.

I met Sheryl many years ago, when I was just a fledgling and beginning my career in the beauty business. She was a very well known makeup artist in a celebrated Beverly Hills salon called The Flamenco. She was also a talented sculptor and painter. This artist applied her talent and skills to bring out the best assets that nature had given to

"It is difficult to be subjected to youth-oriented brainwashing for your entire life and not end up neurotic about turning thirty, forty, fifty, and so on. But life can indeed be wonderful, joyous, and exciting when the bloom of youth turns into the full blossom of maturity."

the women who were fortunate enough to have her use her magic on them; at the same time, she minimized the liabilities that we all have and know so well. The end result would be the emergence of the woman's own natural beauty. Many of her clients would walk out of the salon with one last look in the mirror, feeling like a butterfly just emerging from a cocoon, and these ecstatic women would come back over and over again to learn how my friend Sheryl had recreated them. Step by step she would teach them how to apply their own makeup and show them how to make the most out of what they were born with. She emphasized that in order to look great, a woman should look natural, not heavily made up. Sheryl would say, "The face is like a canvas, and every brush stroke counts." (I would add here that the continued practice of good skin care, as taught in this book, will insure that your canvas is totally clear, clean, and smooth before you begin to do your makeup.)

Sheryl had a quality that went beyond her great ability to transform the physical aspects of these women. She also had the kind of human insight and wisdom needed to encourage their trust. These women would confide in her their most intimate feelings about themselves, sex, love, marriage, their goals in life, their problems—and their fears of the inevitable aging process. Since she was living proof herself of the timelessness of beauty, she was able to reach women on a deeper level. She was able to effect a change in their attitudes regarding femininity, sex appeal, looks, career opportunities, and overall self-image. This makes it sound as if she was a psychotherapist. Well, in many ways she was better. These women, as well as I myself, always trusted her, because her own life reflected the basic truths that she shared:

- that age is an attitude;
- that your inner attitude determines your outward appeal;
- that you can be beautiful at any age;
- that as you get older you have the benefit of being more experienced, more self-confident, more interesting, more fun, more accomplished, smarter, sexier, wiser . . . .

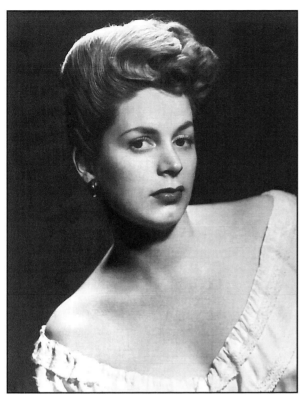

1947

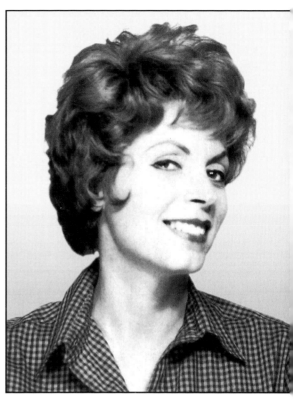

1957

My friend Sheryl—
a beautiful woman
in 1947 (left),
and ten years later,
in 1957.

How's that for starters?

It is important to realize that only in the last two decades have the values of our society started changing in relation to age. Even though the changes have been predominately in society's attitudes toward women, they have also affected men. One of the best indicators of our society's beliefs is what we see on the silver screen. In the not-so-distant past, both actors and actresses were told that there were no leading roles for those over thirty years old. Can you believe that? Today, some of the most romantic roles are being played by gorgeous and interesting leading men and women over thirty, over forty, and over fifty!

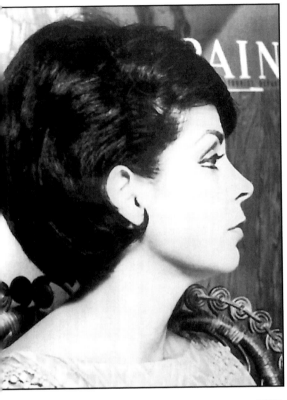

1967

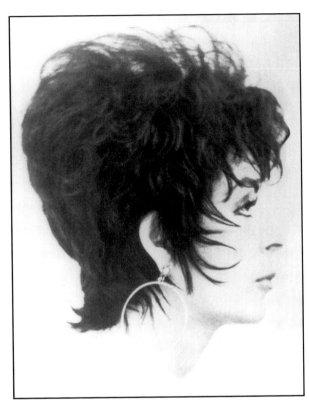

1977

Speaking from my own experience, not only have I been afflicted by the fear of aging, but because I am in the beauty business I have run across many, many women—and also men—who just do not know how to deal with this unchangeable fact of life. You can cure illness, and you can delay death, but you cannot stop the clock from ticking. For this reason, I now want to join with you in exploring this challenge.

First of all, I want to state my frustration about our society's many negative messages regarding aging. It is not news that we are living in an extremely youth-oriented society. As I said earlier, in some areas things have gotten better, such as actors and actresses over

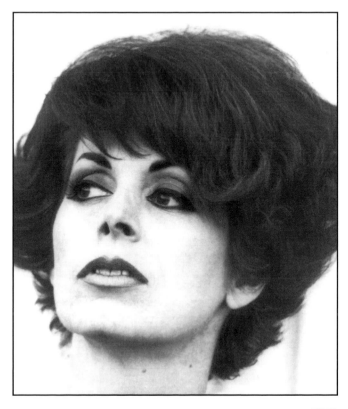

1987

From left: Sheryl in 1967, 1977, and 1987—proof that a woman can be beautiful at any age.

thirty-five or forty finding a wider range of roles open to them. On the other hand, a majority of the media still use the youngest models available for print advertising and television commercials, and to model clothing, hairdos, makeup, skin care products, and so on. These unlined baby faces and perfect size-four bodies are not only a distortion of reality; they also have a real, damaging effect on the psyches of the viewers. Sadly, our society has been driven by the quest for youth. Mindless dieting and plastic surgery have caused many serious mental and physical health problems.

I certainly believe in being lean and healthy, and you know I believe in maintaining great skin and muscle tone throughout the body—but not at the expense of the deeper values we need for a healthy self-image. It is difficult to be subjected to all of this youth-oriented brainwashing for your entire life and not end up being neurotic about turning thirty, forty, fifty, and so on. We just haven't seen a lot of examples of how wonderful, joyous, and exciting life can be when the bloom of youth turns into the full blossom of maturity.

I don't want to paint a completely dark picture, however, because now that the "baby boom" generation has come of age and tremendous numbers of women and men are hitting their mid-forties and fifties, for the first time in history advertising agencies are beginning to use beautiful and interesting older models who have taken great care of themselves and look fabulous. I think it is inspiring for a mature woman to see a woman nearer to her own age acting as a desirable role model. Our society has a long way to go on the subject of age, but at least the doors are starting to open.

This might seem like a contradiction—after all, the name of this book is "Reverse the Aging Process of Your Face." I guess it should really be "Reverse the Aging Process of Your Face *and Mind*." There is absolutely nothing wrong with looking and feeling as good as you can, as long as you live. What is most challenging is, at the same time, to develop the ability to like yourself (or better still, love yourself) at any age.

APPENDIX I

A Glossary of Nature's Bountiful Gifts

The following is a list of ingredients that are often found in the natural cosmetics available in health food stores and that I have found to be most beneficial when used in skin and hair care preparations. There are so many wonderful natural ingredients available, and so much research has been done uncovering their benefits, that this glossary could have turned into a book in itself. However, my main objective is to give you basic information about those ingredients that are the most important and the most commonly used in skin care, hair care, and makeup products. I have chosen to list only those special substances that I know, through my own experience of actually using them in products, have been proven to show the greatest visible benefits to the skin and hair.

If you are interested in further research on this subject, there are several excellent and comprehensive glossaries of natural ingredients available in book and health food stores. There are whole books on the specific categories of enzymes, vitamins, botanicals, herbs, essential oils, aromatherapy, color therapy, and so on. If you are interested in these, consult the bibliography at the end of this book for recommendations.

I have given an individual list of essential oils in Chapter 11, My Unique Approach to Aromatherapy and Color Therapy in Skin Care, in order to separate this field from the larger realm of natural ingredients. Some essential oils are included in this appendix as well. This is because essential oils are used in a somewhat different way and for different reasons when they are incorporated into skin and hair care products.

The ingredients marked with asterisks are very special because they have a twofold benefit: Not only do they beautify the skin and hair, but their use helps to preserve the environment. These are botanicals that are grown in what is called a sustainable yield fashion in the tropical rain forests of the world. This type of production helps to prevent deforestation and promote the survival of the rain forests. I encourage you to purchase products that do not harm our precious earth. For more information on how you can get involved, write or call the Rainforest Action Network (450 Sansome Street, Suite 700, San Francisco, CA 94111; telephone 415-398-4404) and/or Cultural Survival Inc. (215 First Street, Cambridge, MA 02142; telephone 617-621-3818). These are two organizations that I personally have had experience with and whose integrity I believe in.

I hope you enjoy learning about and using these wonderful substances—and also enjoy their results!

*Agave. A botanical from a plant found in tropical and subtropical rain forests. It has moisturizing properties and is soothing to the skin.

Algae. Also known as seaweed, a generic term for a category of more than 20,000 species of mineral-rich plants that live in the sea. Types of algae include marine algae; sea kelp; red, blue, and green algae; bladderwrack; spirulina; and many others. Algae is used a great deal in anti-cellulite products to help eliminate toxins, excess fat, and excess water, and to help purify the skin. Rich in vitamins and useful minerals, algae is used for its moisturizing, firming, and smoothing qualities.

Allantoin. A derivative of the herb comfrey, grown throughout Europe and western Asia, that is known for soothing and smoothing.

*Allspice. An herb grown in the rain forest that is known for soothing the skin.

Almond meal. Finely crushed almonds. Used in Grandma's time and still working for us, almond meal is used in facial and body scrubs to cleanse, massage, and remove dead, dry skin cells.

Aloe vera. A gel-like pulp from inside the leaves of the cactus-type succulent aloe vera plant. Aloe vera has been used at least as far back as ancient Egypt for its extraordinary healing and moisturizing properties. The undiluted gel gives instant relief for burns and sunburns. It is a preferred component in many suntan preparations because of its wonderful soothing and protective qualities, and it is used extensively in a variety of other skin care and cosmetic products for its tremendous soothing, moisturizing, and nourishing benefits.

Alpha-hydroxy acids. A group of acids that are derived from natural sources such as fruits and plants and that have remarkable skin-renewing properties. Alpha-hydroxy acids loosen the chemical bond holding dead, dry skin cells in place, allowing them to be sloughed off and replaced by newer, fresher, healthier cells. This reduces the appearance of fine lines and improves the condition of sun-damaged, mature, or dry skin. Alpha-hydroxy acids also help control oiliness by unblocking oil glands and cleansing the pores. Common types of alpha-hydroxy acids include glycolic acid, lactic acid, malic acid, and bilberry extract.

Alpha-tocopherol. *See* Vitamin E.

Amino acids. Organic compounds that link together to form proteins, amino acids are the basic building blocks of the skin and hair. They are used in skin care treatment products to give a smoother, firmer look and feel to the skin.

Annatto. A yellowish colorant that is sometimes used in natural cosmetics. It is derived from the seeds of a small evergreen shrub that grows in tropical climates.

Antioxidant. Any substance that blocks or retards oxidation reactions. As ingredients in skin care products, they help prevent free radical damage to the skin. Absolutely essential in anti-aging products.

Apricot kernel seeds. A wonderful scrubbing and cleansing agent from the pits of apricots that removes dead skin tissue, stimulates and rejuvenates the skin, and draws out impurities. It leaves a glowing, silky finish to the skin. It is great for sloughing the entire body.

Arnica. A botanical with anti-irritant and astringent qualities. It stimulates circulation and accelerates the removal of wastes from the skin. Arnica is grown in central and southern Europe, central Asia, and North America.

Arrowroot flour. A starch that comes from the roots of a tropical herb and is used as a thickener for foods and also for natural cosmetic products, face and body scrubs, and so on. It can also be used in place of talcum powder.

Avocado oil. A light, not-too-greasy skin nutrient, softener, and conditioner. Avocado oil is noncomedogenic (it does not clog pores).

***Awapuhi.** A botanical grown in the rain forest areas of Hawaii and used in many hair and skin care products for its ability to moisturize, lubricate, and create a sheen.

Azulene. A blue colorant derived from the chamomile flower that is used in many natural skin care and cosmetic products.

***Babassu.** An edible oil derived from the seeds of a tropical palm tree. Also called palm kernel oil, babassu is a very light lubricant and emollient and a great softening agent. It can also be used as a thickening agent.

Balm mint. A plant with skin-soothing and refreshing properties. Grown all over the world.

*Banana oil. A nourishing botanical from the fruit grown in tropical areas. It is used as a skin smoother.

Bee pollen. The microscopic male seed of flowering plants. It is an extremely rich substance with an amazing amount of vitamins, minerals, enzymes, DNA, and RNA, which are very beneficial for the skin.

*Beeswax. A natural wax produced by bees that is used in lip balms, lipsticks, skin creams, hair applications—anywhere a wax is necessary. It should be obtained by sustainable harvesting methods.

Beet juice. An extract from the beet that has a high vitamin and mineral content and is used as a vegetable colorant in natural skin care products.

Bentonite. An absorbent mineral clay that is very healing, soothing, detoxifying, and rich in minerals. It is used in masks and makeup products.

Benzoic acid. An antiseptic used to control acne. It occurs naturally in cherry bark, raspberries, anise, and cassia bark. It is found in many over-the-counter acne products.

Benzophene-3. A sunscreen that blocks the sun's ultraviolet-A (UVA) rays. It is a synthetic organic compound.

Beta-carotene. *See* Vitamin A.

Beta-glucan. A substance derived from yeast and oats that is used in skin care products for its soothing qualities. It has been shown to smooth lines and even out skin texture. It is also sometimes called modified oat flour.

Beta-hydroxy acid. A term used to refer to salicylic acid, benzoic acid, buteric acid, and a number of other, less well known acids. These substances have been used for many years in over-the-counter acne products, but are now classified as beta-hydroxy acids. They are similar to alpha-hydroxy acids in their action, but they have a slightly different chemical structure. Like alpha-hydroxy acids, they have the effect of exfoliating the skin.

Bilberry extract. A source of alpha-hydroxy acids, or fruit acid extracts.

Bioflavonoids. Biologically active substances, derived principally from fruits, that are important for maintaining the health of blood vessel walls. They are also powerful antioxidants and anti-aging factors that stimulate collagen production. Associated with vitamin C, bioflavonoids are often used in skin care products for their astringent, cleansing, and skin-refining properties.

Biotin. A member of the B-vitamin family used in many hair care products to strengthen the hair follicles, hair shafts, and scalp. It is also said to help hair growth and make hair thicker.

Bladderwrack. A plant grown in coastal regions that contains many of the minerals found in seaweed, algae, and other plants from the sea.

Borage oil. Oil from the herb borage, a natural botanical that has a high percentage of antioxidants, gamma-linolenic acid (GLA), and unsaturated fatty acids ("vitamin F").

*Brazil nut oil. A lubricant from the rain forests and tropical areas. It helps smooth and maintain the elasticity of the skin.

Bromelain. An enzyme from the pineapple fruit. It is very good for all skin types, especially for oily or acne-prone skin.

Calendula. A purifying botanical that softens, soothes, and helps minimize puffiness. It also has antioxidant properties.

Camphor. A natural extract from the camphor tree that is used for its antiseptic and anti-inflammatory effects.

Candelilla wax. A natural wax derived from the candelilla plant that acts as an emollient. It is used in lipsticks, lip glosses, and solid powders to give body to the product and lubrication to the skin.

Canola oil. A natural vegetable oil that is an excellent replacement for mineral oil due to its similar viscosity and great lubricity. It is also sometimes called rapeseed oil.

Capsicum extract. Extract of cayenne pepper. Used in skin care and massage preparations, it stimulates circulation and warms up muscles.

*Carnauba wax. A wax from the leaves of the Brazilian wax palm tree that is used in virtually all lipsticks and lip glosses, and many make-up products.

Castor oil. An oil derived from the seeds of the castor-oil plant. It soothes, moisturizes, and lubricates the skin, and is used in many makeup products, including lipsticks, lip glosses, and foundation.

Cayenne. *See* Capsicum extract.

Chamomile. A botanical that acts as an antioxidant and is used to help relieve inflammation and soothe skin. Chamomile oil is very popular in aromatherapy.

Citric acid. An acid that is found in citrus fruits and that is rich in vitamin C, a powerful antioxidant.

Clay. There are many types and colors of this mineral-rich earth substance from all over the world. Also sometimes referred to as mud, it dissolves dead skin cells, absorbs impurities, helps reduce enlarged pores, and gives the skin a firmer look and texture. Also helps to heal burns and abrasions and to relieve swelling.

*Cocoa butter. A buttery substance derived from cocoa beans that is used for sun protection and lubrication.

*Coconut oil. An oil from the fruit of the coconut tree, grown in tropical and rain forest areas. It is an excellent moisturizer that serves as a protective layer to hold moisture in the skin. It also gives great lubricity to skin care products.

*Cohune oil. Oil from a nut grown in the Guatemalan rain forest. It is an elegant, light emollient oil with a soft, pleasing feel on the skin.

Collagen. A fibrous protein that helps to uphold and nourish the cellular structure of the skin.

Comfrey. An herb grown throughout Europe and western Asia. It is known for its soothing and smoothing properties.

Coneflower. *See* Echinacea.

*Copaiba. A botanical from tropical South American rain forests that is a healing antiseptic and has antioxidant properties.

Corn flour. *See* Cornmeal.

Cornmeal. The ground meal from the cob of the corn. Also referred to as corn flour, it is an excellent exfoliator, or sloughing agent, that is very beneficial in scrubs.

Cucumber. A botanical that tightens pores, softens rough skin, refreshes, soothes, and moisturizes. Whole cucumber slices placed on the eyes help to relieve puffiness and swelling.

Dimethicone. Derived from silica (from ground, micronized sand), dimethicone is used in many cosmetic products for the silky smooth look and feel it gives to the skin.

DNA and RNA. Nucleic acids (deoxyribonucleic acid and ribonucleic acid), the material found inside the cells that contains the cells' genetic "code." Both DNA and RNA must be protected from destruction caused by invasive free radicals. The use of antioxidants, both externally and internally, is vitally important. DNA and RNA can be derived from yeast and used in skin care products to replenish and reinforce DNA and RNA in the layers of the skin.

d-Panthenol. *See* Panthenol.

Echinacea. A softening and soothing botanical, excellent for relaxing and refreshing the eye area. It is also sometimes referred to as coneflower.

EFA. *See* Essential fatty acids.

Elastin. A protein that is part of the network of the skin, along with collagen. It works with collagen to nourish and uphold the skin tissue.

Elder flower. An anti-inflammatory, cleansing botanical that helps to minimize pores and soothe skin.

Emollient. A general term used for all lubricants that soothe, soften, and nourish the skin. Emollients are an absolute necessity for preventing and correcting dry skin.

Emulsifier. An agent necessary to mix oil and water together. Emulsifiers are used in virtually all cosmetic creams and lotions.

Ergocalciferol. *See* Vitamin D.

Essential fatty acids (EFAs). Elements found in all natural vegetable oils that are vitally necessary for keeping skin healthy, soft, enriched, and smooth. They are also sometimes referred to as "vitamin F."

Eucalyptus oil. Oil derived from the leaves of the eucalyptus tree. It is used for its antiseptic and stimulant properties; it is also used frequently as a decongestant and detoxifier. It is very popular with aromatherapists.

Evening primrose oil. A skin smoother, rich in nutrients, derived from the evening primrose plant. It is very high in gamma-linolenic acid, an essential fatty acid that is needed for very smooth and healthy skin.

Fatty esters. Chains of natural oil molecules. Fatty esters give a great lubricity and smoothing texture to the skin. They are used in many skin care products.

Fennel. A botanical often used to fight inflammation.

Free radicals. Highly reactive molecules, atoms, or ions that can be destructive if they attack healthy cells and damage their nucleic acids (DNA and RNA), causing premature aging and damage to the immune system. Free radical activity can also lead to serious skin damage.

Gamma-linolenic acid (GLA). An essential fatty acid derived from natural vegetable oil sources that is used in many skin care products. It is necessary for lubrication and nourishment of the skin and, internally, of the body as a whole.

Gentian root. A botanical used for its astringent properties.

Geranium. A flowering plant that has anti-inflammatory and soothing properties.

Germanium. A trace element that is a strong immune-system strengthener, antioxidant, and free-radical fighter. Natural botanicals that are rich in germanium include suma and ginseng.

Ginkgo biloba. A botanical that comes from the Far East and contains powerful antioxidants known for their anti-aging properties. It helps to protect skin from damaging free radicals and also improves circulation, for a healthier body and healthier, rosy, younger looking skin.

Ginseng. A well-known Asian herb that is acclaimed as an antioxidant and immune-system strengthener. It is rejuvenating, oxygenating, and stimulating for the skin and entire body. It has also been said to strengthen the skin surface, to make skin more resilient, and to help balance the production of needed natural lipids.

GLA. *See* Gamma-linolenic acid.

Glycerin. A commonly used moisturizer and emollient derived from vegetable fats.

Glycolic acid. An alpha-hydroxy acid derived from sugar cane. It was the first of the alpha-hydroxy acids to be highly acclaimed, because dermatologists used it for deep skin peels.

Goldenseal. A native American herb that is known to strengthen the immune system. It is used for its detoxifying and anti-inflammatory qualities.

Grapefruit seed extract. An extract with excellent cleansing and anti-inflammatory qualities. It is also very high in citric acid and is used to help preserve skin care products.

Henna. A dye derived from the leaves of a small tree or shrub (*Lawsonia inermis*) native to the Middle East. The world's oldest natural hair coloring agent and conditioner (its use dates at least as far back as the ancient Egyptian queen Nefertiti), henna has made a comeback as a natural alternative to chemical hair dyes.

*Honey. Honey has wonderful healing properties and aids in drawing out impurities when used in scrubs and masks.

Horsetail. A botanical used for soothing, smoothing, and moisturizing skin.

Humectant. Another word for a moisturizer. Humectants are used to preserve the moisture content of the skin as well as to draw moisture from the air and direct it to the skin.

Hyaluronic acid. *See* Sodium hyaluronate.

Irish moss. A sea botanical, also sometimes referred to as sea moss, known for its purifying properties, used to help heal skin breakouts and reduce cellulite. *See also* Algae.

*Jaboncillo berry. A fruity botanical extract from the rain forest that is known for its astringent properties.

Jojoba oil. A botanical oil that has been used for centuries by Native Americans as a scalp tonic. Research has shown that this waxy extract of the jojoba seed can remove the embedded sebum deposits around hair follicles that can cause dandruff, hair loss, and weakening of the hair structure. Many people have claimed that jojoba oil renews hair growth when used as a scalp cleanser/massage oil, even in cases of balding or excessive thinning of the hair. Jojoba oil is now used in many skin care and makeup products for its great moisturizing and lubricating qualities.

Kaolin. A fine, mineral-rich clay known for its soothing, detoxifying, and skin-firming benefits. It is used in masks and many makeup products.

Keratin. A protein that is the chief component of hair. It is used in hair care products because it can penetrate into the hair shaft, where it works to rebuild and repair damaged hair and split ends. Keratin is often combined with panthenol in shampoo and conditioner formulas.

*Kukui nut. This rain forest botanical is rich in an oil that is known for soothing and softening the skin.

Lactic acid. An alpha-hydroxy acid derived from substances such as sour milk and bilberry extract. A combination of lactic and glycolic acid has been shown to be more effective for skin rejuvenation than glycolic acid alone.

Lecithin. A substance classified as a phospholipid that is one of the most important natural moisturizing agents, because of its good compatibility with the skin and its ability to penetrate into the skin. It is rich in unsaturated fatty acids. When used in creams, its emollient properties keep skin plumped up, soft, supple, and youthful-looking. Lecithin is also employed as the outer shell of liposomes. Most lecithin is obtained from soybeans.

Lemon peel. A natural detoxifying astringent that is high in citric acid and vitamin C. It is used for both its cleansing properties and its wonderful natural fragrance.

Lemongrass. A cleansing and purifying botanical that is rich in vitamin C and has great astringent qualities.

Licorice extract. An anti-irritant and anti-inflammatory that is used in skin care products for its soothing qualities.

Linden. A botanical produced primarily in Switzerland and elsewhere in northern Europe. It is used for its skin-smoothing and softening properties.

Liposomes. Microscopic spheres used in skin care products to deliver active ingredients to the skin cells. This highly advanced delivery system can significantly enhance the performance of the transported ingredients because it can more effectively penetrate the skin. Look for products containing liposomes made with and containing natural ingredients.

Macadamia nut oil. An oil rich in nutrients that are very soothing and smoothing to the skin.

Magnesium aluminum silicate. A naturally occurring earth mineral that is used as a thickener in skin care and makeup products.

Malic acid. An alpha-hydroxy acid that is derived from a variety of sources, including apples and the sugar maple tree. It is used in many alpha-hydroxy acid products.

Marsh mallow. An emollient herb that is used as a soothing skin softener in many creams and lotions.

Menthol. A derivative of peppermint, spearmint, or any mint oil. Menthol is used for cleansing and stimulating the skin. One of the most cooling, refreshing, and invigorating natural substances from the plant world, it is also used to ease aching muscles.

Menthyl lactate. A cooling agent derived from menthol.

Methylparaben and propylparaben. Preservatives used to protect skin care and cosmetic products from bacterial growth and dangerous contamination. They are derived from a botanical, gum benzoin, and have been used successfully and safely for many years.

Milk protein. A good source of amino acids and lactic acid (one of the alpha-hydroxy acids). When used in creams and lotions, milk protein helps to repair, smooth, and strengthen skin tissue.

Milk thistle. A botanical with powerful antioxidant qualities that is used as a skin detoxifier. Taken internally, milk thistle has been shown to benefit the liver and help correct liver damage. It helps to improve the functioning of the immune system externally as well as internally. It is also called silymarin.

Mucopolysaccharides. A basic component of skin tissue that surrounds the elastin and collagen fibers and provides the environment needed to make these proteins work efficiently. Mucopolysaccharides act as a lubricating agent for the support of the connective tissue and mucous membranes.

Mud. *See* Clay.

NaPCA. A natural protein that is known to dramatically attract and hold on to moisture in the skin. It is used frequently in toners, astringents, and gel-type formulas. Also called sodium PCA.

Nettle. A soothing, detoxifying botanical.

Oak bark. An herb known for its natural astringent and skin-firming qualities.

Oat flour. *See* Beta-glucan.

Octyl methoxycinnamate. A sunscreen that blocks the sun's ultraviolet-B (UVB) rays. It oxygenates, protects, and guards the skin against harmful rays and environmental toxins. It is derived from cinnamon and cassia oil.

Olive oil unsaponifiable. *See* Squalane.

Orange peel extract. A botanical that has an astringent effect and has been found to be very beneficial for cellulite problems. It has a high concentration of citric acid. It is also used for its wonderful fragrance.

*Orchid oil. An oil from the tropical orchid plant that contributes softening and moisturizing qualities to skin care products.

Palm kernel oil. *See* Babassu.

Panthenol. A vitamin precursor that is well received by the skin and hair, and has skin- and hair-strengthening properties. Laboratory tests have shown its great restorative properties for both hair and skin. When used in shampoos and hair rinses, it can thicken hair volume up to 10 percent and help mend damaged hair. It is also healing and soothing for many kinds of skin disorders and irritations. It is an important addition to all cosmetic products for its nourishing, enlivening benefits. It may also be referred to as d-panthenol, dl-panthenol, or pro-vitamin B_5.

Papaya extract. A fruit extract that contains the enzyme papain, which absorbs and dissolves dead, dry surface skin cells and helps condition the skin. Great when used in scrubs and masks.

Passion flower. A skin-detoxifying tropical botanical used for reducing inflammation and soothing the skin.

Peach kernel oil. A vegetable oil rich in unsaturated fatty acids, which are important for proper lubrication of the skin. It is used in many natural skin creams and lotions.

Peach kernel seeds. Like apricot kernel seeds, these make for wonderful scrubbing and cleansing agents that remove dead skin tissue and stimulate, rejuvenate, and draw out impurities from the skin, leaving a healthy, glowing, and silky texture. A great abrasive treatment for exfoliating the entire body.

pH balance. The correct balance between acidity and alkalinity. To keep skin and hair in utmost health, the pH of any skin or hair care product should be similar to the body's own natural pH, between 5.0 and 7.0.

Plantain extract. A botanical extract that has astringent properties and helps to draw out toxins and reduce fatty deposits (cellulite).

Propylparaben. *See* Methylparaben.

Pycnogenol. A powerful antioxidant derived from the bark of the North American anneda pine tree.

Pyruvic acid. An alpha-hydroxy acid derived from citrus fruits.

Rapeseed oil. *See* Canola oil.

Retin-A. A brand-name prescription product containing tretinoin, a member of the vitamin-A family. It is used to improve the appearance of aging skin by causing a peeling of the skin and sloughing off of dead cells, as well as a plumping up of thinning and wrinkled skin. It also makes skin very vulnerable to sunburn and sun damage.

Retinol. *See* Vitamin A.

Retinyl palmitate. *See* Vitamin A.

RNA. *See* DNA.

Rosa mosqueta. An oil derived from the hips of a wild rose grown in Chile. Rich in vitamin C and essential fatty acids known for their healing properties, it helps preserve the texture and feel of young skin.

Rose hips. The fruit of the rose plant. Rose hip extract is rich in vitamin C, a powerful antioxidant and anti-aging component that helps to preserve skin from destructive elements. It also helps to prevent the breakdown of collagen.

Rosemary. A stimulating, tonic herb known to aid in hair growth, conditioning, and scalp regeneration. It is one of the most effective components of any great scalp massage preparation. It can also be mixed with any oil to make an excellent massage oil for aching muscles and to promote circulation.

Royal bee jelly. A gift direct from her highness, the queen bee, royal jelly is a soluble substance that is rich in vitamins, minerals, and protein, and creates a younger, smoother looking skin.

Rye flour. A whole-grain flour that is used in many scrubs for its great cleansing and abrasive qualities.

Safflower oil. A rich but noncomedogenic (non-pore-clogging) vegetable oil that is used to moisturize and lubricate the skin.

Sage extract. An extract from the sage plant that is used for its astringent, stimulating, and tonic properties.

Salicylic acid. A naturally occurring acid (found in wintergreen leaves, sweet birch, and other plants) that acts as an exfoliant. It is also sometimes referred to as beta-hydroxy acid. Unlike alpha-hydroxy acids, which unglue the bond that attaches dead, dry surface skin cells to the skin that lies beneath, salicylic acid exfoliates the top layer of skin (the stratum corneum). It is used in many over-the-counter acne preparations because of its potent antibacterial and antiseptic qualities.

*Sapayul. A great nutrient botanical extract for skin and scalp. It is grown in the rain forests.

Sea kelp. A sea plant that is highly effective for cleansing, exfoliating, and regenerating the skin tissue. Used in scrubs, this effective ingredient deep cleanses, smooths, and helps clear up skin eruptions. One of my all-time favorite ingredients.

Sea moss. *See* Irish moss.

Sea salt. A very effective purifying and sloughing ingredient. It is great when combined with sea kelp in all types of exfoliating products.

Seaweed. *See* Algae.

Selenium. A trace mineral and antioxidant that combats damaging free radicals and helps strengthen the immune system.

Sesame oil. The oil from the sesame seed. It is known for its high concentration of essential fatty acids, which are great for smoothing and lubricating the skin.

Shea butter. A rich, buttery vegetable oil from the African karite nut tree. It has special skin-enriching properties that give a glowing, youthful look to the skin.

Silymarin. *See* Milk thistle.

Skin respiratory factor (SRF). *See* Tissue respiratory factor.

SOD. *See* Superoxide dismutase.

Sodium hyaluronate. A powerful humectant that has the ability to attract moisture from the air and bind that water to skin tissue for a long period of time. This contributes to the skin's elasticity and suppleness, and minimizes the appearance of lines and wrinkles by plumping up the skin. Sodium hyaluronate is created from a long chain of molecules derived from glucose. Also known as hyaluronic acid.

Sodium PCA. *See* NaPCA.

Soybean oil. A natural vegetable oil with excellent absorbing and moisturizing properties. It is used in many natural cosmetics.

Soy lecithin. *See* Lecithin.

Spanish juniper. A stimulant and anti-irritant derived from a berry grown in Europe, northern Asia, and North Africa.

SPF. *See* Sun protection factor.

Squalane. A source of natural fatty acids and one of the highest grade lubricants in skin care products. It is used to help increase skin respiration and prevent the loss of moisture. It helps retard the signs of premature aging. Unlike its predecessor, squalene, which came from animal sources, squalane is a vegetable-based product. Also sometimes referred to as olive oil unsaponifiable.

SRF. *See* Tissue respiratory factor.

*Suma. A botanical from the tropical forests of Brazil that helps to balance and smooth skin. It is rich in antioxidants and provides an amazing amount of vitamins, minerals, and other nutrients to help fight free radicals and retard aging.

Sun protection factor (SPF). A measurement of the effectiveness of sunscreens and sun blocks. The SPF number refers to how many times longer than normal a product will allow you to be out in the sun without getting burned.

Superoxide dismutase (SOD). A nutrient enzyme derived from yeast that is one of the best known antioxidants. It helps protect skin from toxins and free radicals, and stimulates the production of collagen.

Tartaric acid. An alpha-hydroxy acid found in grapes.

Thyme. A very popular herb used for its anti-inflammatory but stimulating and conditioning properties. Also called wild thyme.

Tissue respiratory factor (TRF). An anti-aging protein derived from yeast that is used for its skin-smoothing and cell-renewal abilities. It acts as an anti-inflammatory, and when used in a liposome, its moisturizing benefits can be delivered over a longer period of time as well as more efficiently to the skin's surface. Also called skin respiratory factor (SRF).

Titanium dioxide. A nontoxic protective compound used for years in makeup and skin care products. It imparts opacity to makeup and is now used as a sunscreen and sun block as well. It reflects light rather than absorbing it. It is listed on many product labels as TiO_2.

Tocopheryl acetate. *See* Vitamin E.

TRF. *See* Tissue respiratory factor.

*Vanilla bean. A botanical originally derived from the rain forests of Mexico. It is used in many skin care and fragrance products for its soothing, uplifting effects on both the skin and the senses.

Vegetable oils. Oils derived from plant sources. Beneficial, non-comedogenic vegetable oils include apricot kernel, almond, avocado, borage, canola, carrot, coconut, evening primrose, jojoba, olive, peach kernel, peanut, rice bran, safflower, sesame, soy, sunflower, and wheat germ oils, among others. There are also many great oils derived from rain forest plants, such as Brazil nut, kukui nut, babassu (palm kernel), copaiba, banana, sapayul, cohune, and others that are sustainably harvested. All of these oils are rich in unsaturated fatty acids, vitamins, and minerals that are important for superior lubrication of the skin tissue.

Vegetable protein. Soluble and hydrolyzed proteins from wheat, soy, marine plants, and other vegetable sources that help to uphold and nourish the cellular structure of the skin. These are highly sophisticated substitutes that are directly comparable in molecular structure to animal proteins, such as elastin and collagen, that are used in cosmetics and skin care products.

Vitamin A. A family of compounds that includes beta-carotene and retinyl palmitate. Vitamin A is a fat-soluble vitamin that nourishes and revitalizes the skin, increases skin elasticity, and helps to regenerate skin cells, thereby decreasing lines and creating healthier, more supple looking skin. It is also a potent antioxidant that is used to protect skin tissue and cells from damaging free radicals, especially those caused by exposure to the sun's ultraviolet rays. Also called retinol.

Vitamin C. A renowned antioxidant that also upholds and improves the functioning of the capillaries that feed the skin. Used in skin care preparations, it has been shown to speed up regeneration of collagen-producing fibroblasts; there is also evidence that it helps to repair skin damage done by the sun. It shows great power when combined with vitamin E in anti-aging research.

Vitamin D. Once called the "sunshine vitamin," vitamin D has been added to skin creams for many years for its smoothing and anti-aging properties. It is often used in combination with vitamin A for skin smoothing. It is sometimes also referred to as ergocalciferol.

Vitamin E. A powerful anti-aging free-radical fighter (antioxidant) and skin rejuvenator. Vitamin E helps to soothe and heal dry, burned, and sun-damaged skin; it lubricates and enriches any skin, helps increase the amount of oxygen present in skin cells, and promotes the growth of healthy tissue. It also helps minimize stretch marks if used regularly during pregnancy. Research shows it becomes an even more powerful antioxidant when used in combination with vitamin C.

Vitamin E may also appear on labels as alpha-tocopheryl or tocopheryl acetate.

Vitamin F. *See* Essential fatty acids.

Walnut shells. A wonderful natural ingredient used in many exfoliating scrubs. Ground walnut shells are very purifying, detoxifying, and satinizing for the skin of the face and all over the body.

Wheat germ oil. An oil rich in vitamin E that has free-radical-fighting qualities. It is very well absorbed and has excellent moisturizing and skin-rejuvenating properties.

Wild thyme. *See* Thyme.

Witch hazel. An herb that is both astringent and soothing.

Yarrow. An herb known for its skin-stimulating properties.

Yeast. Tiny single-celled organisms that are loaded with B vitamins and protein, as well as many other skin nutrients. This food substance has a very stimulating effect when used in facial masks. It boosts blood circulation in skin tissue when used topically.

Zinc oxide. A compound of the mineral zinc that is used in makeup, sun care, and skin care products. It imparts opacity to makeup and also is used as an astringent and protectant. It is believed to encourage healing of skin disorders.

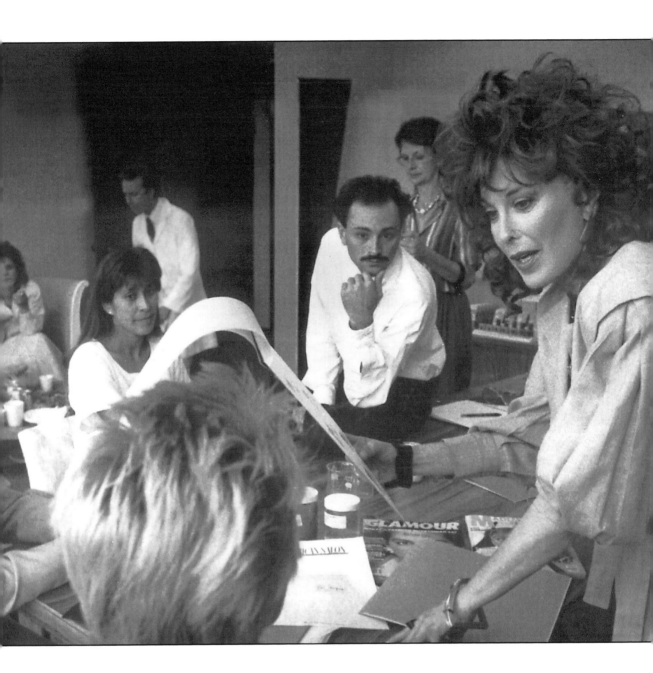

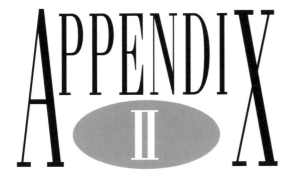

APPENDIX II

A Guide to Rachel Perry Products

This section contains a list of Rachel Perry skin care products, classified according to product type and the type of skin for which they are appropriate. All of my products are designed for use with my facial exercise and massage technique. They are available at cosmetic boutiques, beauty outlets, and better natural foods shops throughout the United States, Canada, and internationally.

CLEANSERS

Normal and Combination Skin
  Citrus-Aloe Cleanser & Face Wash
  Tangerine Dream Foaming Facial Cleanser With
    Alpha-Hydroxy Acids
Dry, Very Dry, and Aging Skin
  Citrus-Aloe Cleanser & Face Wash
Oily or Acne-Prone Skin
  Tangerine Dream Foaming Facial Cleanser With
    Alpha-Hydroxy Acids

Sensitive Skin
   Citrus-Aloe Cleanser & Face Wash
   Tangerine Dream Foaming Facial Cleanser With
      Alpha-Hydroxy Acids

EXFOLIATORS

Normal and Combination Skin
   Sea Kelp-Herbal Facial Scrub
   Peach & Papaya Gentle Facial Scrub
Dry, Very Dry, and Aging Skin
   Sea Kelp-Herbal Facial Scrub
   Peach & Papaya Gentle Facial Scrub
Oily or Acne-Prone Skin
   Sea Kelp-Herbal Facial Scrub
   Peach & Papaya Gentle Facial Scrub
Sensitive Skin
   Peach & Papaya Gentle Facial Scrub
   Dilute with water if skin is extra sensitive.

MASKS (ALL SKIN TYPES)

   Clay & Ginseng Texturizing Mask

TONERS

Normal Skin
   Violet-Rose Skin Toner
Combination Skin
   Violet-Rose Skin Toner (for cheek area)
   Lemon-Mint Astringent (for T-zone)
Dry, Very Dry, and Aging Skin
   Violet-Rose Skin Toner

Oily or Acne-Prone Skin
  Lemon-Mint Astringent
  Perfectly Clear Herbal Antiseptic
Sensitive Skin
  Violet-Rose Skin Toner

FIRMING TREATMENT (ALL SKIN TYPES)

Vegetable "Elastin & Collagen" Firming Treatment

MOISTURIZERS

Normal and Combination Skin
  Lecithin-Aloe Moisture Retention Cream
  Calendula-Cucumber Oil Free Moisturizer
  For best results, use both, but on alternating days.
Dry, Very Dry, and Aging Skin
  Bee Pollen-Jojoba Maximum Moisture Cream
  Lecithin-Aloe Moisture Rentention Cream
  For best results, use both, but on alternating days.
Oily or Acne-Prone Skin
  Calendula-Cucumber Oil Free Moisturizer
Sensitive Skin
  Lecithin-Aloe Moisture Retention Cream
  Bee Pollen-Jojoba Maximum Moisture Cream
  For best results, use both, but on alternating days.

NOURISHING CREAMS (ALL SKIN TYPES)

Hi-Potency "E" Special Treatment Line Control (16,000 IU)
Ginseng & Vegetable "Collagen" Wrinkle Treatment With
  High Potency C
For best results, use both, but on alternating days. For combination skin, use on dry areas and neck only; for oily or acne-prone skin, use around the eyes and possibly on neck (if dry) only.

163

SPECIAL TREATMENTS (ALL SKIN TYPES)

*Immediately Visible Eye Renewal Gel-Cream
    With Liposomes
Visible Transition Alpha-Hydroxy Serum*

LIP CARE (ALL SKIN TYPES)

Lip Lover moisturizing lip balm with sunscreen

BODY CARE (ALL SKIN TYPES)

*Rainforest Botanical Therapy Shower and Bath Gel
Rainforest Botanical Therapy Body Lotion
Sea & Earth French Massage Formula
Sea & Earth Spearmint Leaf Body Scrub
Sea & Earth Spearmint Leaf Body Wash
Sea & Earth Spearmint Leaf Revitalizing Body
    Lotion*

NATURAL NUTRIENT MAKEUP COLLECTION

Makeup
   *Bee Pollen-Jojoba Nutrient Makeup Foundation
   Chamomile Translucent Powder
   Jojoba Secret Cover*
Blush
   *Chamomile Radiant Blushing Powder
   Earth Blush Cream*
Eye Fashions
   *Vegetable "Elastin-Collagen" Eyeshadow
   Nutrient Automatic Eyeliner Pencil
   Vegetable "Elastin-Collagen" Lash Building Mascara
   Evening Primrose Oil Eye Makeup Remover*

Lip Collection
  Nutrient Luster Lipstick
  Nutrient Automatic Lip Liner Pencil
  Nutrient Luster Lip Gloss

NOTES

Chapter 1
A Simple Technique That Works

1. Frederick M. Rossiter, *Face Culture* (New York: Pageant Press Inc., 1956).

Chapter 4
Moisturizing and Nourishing a Thirsty, Hungry Skin

1. Brian C. Keller, BioZone Laboratories, Inc., personal communication, August 1994.

Chapter 7
The Sun: Friend or Foe?

1. Peter Pugliese, "Sun And Your Client," *Skin Inc.*, July 1990, 60.

Chapter 8
Skin Fitness for the Body Beautiful

1. "On Marketing Youth," *Longevity*, June 1993, 69.
2. Ibid, 73.
3. *Dermascope*, July/August 1994.
4. Brian C. Keller, BioZone Laboratories, Inc., personal communication, August 1994.

BIBLIOGRAPHY

Abehsera, Michael. *The Healing Clay: Ancient Treatments for Modern Times*. Brooklyn, NY: Swan House Publishing Company, 1977.

"Alpha Hydroxy Acid Skin Peels and the FDA." CBS news report, 24 October 1994.

American Academy of Dermatology. "Alpha Hydroxy Acids Reduce Wrinkles." News release. Chicago: American Academy of Dermatology, 15 September 1987.

"Aminophylline." CNN news report, 23 October 1993.

"Aminophylline." NBC news report, 4 November 1993.

Anderson, Mary. *Colour Healing*. New York: Samuel Wiser Inc, 1975.

Berman, Michael, and Sharon Flynn. "Renewable Rainforest Resources." *Drug and Cosmetic Industry*, Vol. 156 (February 1995).

Birren, Faber. *Color in Your World*. New York: Crowell-Collier Publishing, 1962.

Birren, Faber. *Color Psychology and Color Therapy.* Secaucus, NJ: University Books Inc., 1961.

Blumenthal, Mark. *HerbalGram: The Journal of the American Botanical Council and the Herb Research Foundation,* No. 7 (Fall 1985).

——— *HerbalGram: The Journal of the American Botanical Council and the Herb Research Foundation,* No. 11 (Winter 1987).

——— *HerbalGram: The Journal of the American Botanical Council and the Herb Research Foundation,* No. 16 (Spring 1988).

——— *HerbalGram: The Journal of the American Botanical Council and the Herb Research Foundation,* No. 20 (Spring 1989).

——— *HerbalGram: The Journal of the American Botanical Council and the Herb Research Foundation,* No. 21 (Fall 1989).

——— *HerbalGram: The Journal of the American Botanical Council and the Herb Research Foundation,* No. 22 (Spring 1990).

——— *HerbalGram: The Journal of the American Botanical Council and the Herb Research Foundation,* No. 25 (Summer 1991).

——— *HerbalGram: The Journal of the American Botanical Council and the Herb Research Foundation,* No. 33 (Spring 1995).

Clark, Linda. *The Ancient Art of Color Therapy.* New York: Pocket Books, 1978.

Clark, Linda, and Yvonne Martine. *Health, Youth and Beauty Through Color Breathing.* Millbrae, CA: Celestial Arts Publishing, 1976.

de Franco, V. James. "Summary Report and Panel Study of Topical Fat Reduction Formula." Pittsburg, CA: BioZone Laboratories Inc., July 1994.

Djerassi, David, Lawrence J. Machlin, and Carlor Nocka. "Vitamin E Biochemical Function and Its Role in Cosmetics." *Drug and Cosmetic Industry,* March 1986.

Duke, James A. "Actiphyte (R) of Japanese Green Tea Concentrate." *Active Organics: Handbook of Medicinal Herbs.* Boca Raton, FL: CRC Press Inc., 1985.

"Ethocyn Treatment." CBS news report, 3 August 1994.

Flippin, Royce. "Battle of the Bulges." *American Health*, January/February 1993.

Fox, Charles. "Innovative Ingredients." *Skin Inc.*, September 1991.

Gadberry, Rebecca James. "Thigh-Buster Creams: Getting the Skinny on Fat's Latest Fad." *Dermascope*, July/August 1994.

Godfrey-June, Jean. "The AHA Phenomenon." Interview with Lawrence Moy, M.D. *Longevity*, September 1993.

Grieve, M. *A Modern Herbal*, Vol. 2. New York: Dover Publications Inc., 1971.

Hirsch, Alan. "Aromatherapy Scent Inhalers for Weight Loss." CNN news report, 18 June 1994.

Hirsch, Alan. "Aromatherapy Scent Inhalers for Weight Loss." NBC news report, 12 September 1994.

Howard, Rebecca. "Acid and Facial Creams." Interview with Lawrence Moy, M.D. *LA Life*, 4 February 1993.

Jouhar, A.J., ed. *Poucher's Perfumes, Cosmetics and Soaps*, 9th ed. Vol. 1, *The Raw Materials of Perfumery*, by W.A. Poucher. London, England: Chapman and Hall, 1991.

―――― *Poucher's Perfumes, Cosmetics and Soaps*, 9th ed. Vol. 2, *The Production, Manufacture and Application of Perfumes*, by W.A. Poucher. London, England: Chapman and Hall, 1991.

―――― *Poucher's Perfumes, Cosmetics and Soaps*, 9th ed. Vol. 3, *Cosmetics*, by W.A. Poucher. London, England: Chapman and Hall, 1991.

Lavabre, Marcel F. *The Handbook of Aromatherapy, or How to Cure Yourself*. Culver City, CA: Marcel F. Lavabre Publishing, Inc., 1986.

Luscher, Max. *The Luscher Color Test*. New York: Random House Inc., 1969.

Margales, Miguel. "An Active Complex for Prevention of Skin Aging." *Drug and Cosmetic Industry*, September 1992.

Morris, Edwin T. *Fragrance: The Story of Perfume From Cleopatra to Chanel*. New York: Charles Scribner's Sons, 1984.

Moy, Lawrence S. "Measurable Effects of the Liposome Fat Contour Cream." In *Liposome Technology*, edited by Gregory Gregoriadis. Boca Raton, FL: CRC Press, 1993.

Murad, Howard, and Paul Scott Premo. "A Primer on Glycolic Acid." *Dermascope*, April 1993.

"On Marketing Youth." *Longevity*, June 1993.

Newman, Arnold. *Tropical Rainforest*. New York: Facts on File, 1990.

Ousley, S.G.J. *Color Meditations*. Essex, England: L.N. Fowler & Co., Ltd., 1990.

Packer, Lester. "Vitamin E, Physical Exercise, and Tissue Oxidative Damage, Biology of Vitamin E." Ciba Foundation Symposium 101, 1983.

Phelps-Brown, O. *The Complete Herbalist*. North Hollywood, CA: Newcastle Publishing Company, 1993.

"Pheromones and DHEA." CBS news report, 12 May 1994.

Pugliese, Peter. *Advanced Professional Skin Care*. Bernville, PA: APSC Publishing, 1991.

Silcock, Lisa, Ed. *The Rainforests—A Celebration*. San Francisco: Chronicle Books, 1990.

Pugliese, Peter. "Sun and Your Client." *Skin Inc.*, July 1990.

Smith, Walter. "Hydroxy Acids With Skin Aging." *Soap/Cosmetics/ Chemical Specialties*, September 1993.

Thie, John F. *Touch for Health*. Pasadena, CA: T.H. Enterprises, 1987.

Tisserand, Maggie. *Aromatherapy for Women*. Rochester, VT: Healing Arts Press, 1985.

Tisserand, Robert. *Aromatherapy: To Heal and Tend the Body*. Santa Fe, NM: C.W. Daniel Company, Ltd., 1988.

Wilson, Roberta. *Aromatherapy for Vibrant Health and Beauty*. Garden City Park, NY: Avery Publishing Group, 1995.

Wren, R.C. *Potter's New Cyclopaedia of Botanical Drugs and Preparations*, revised by Elizabeth M. Williamson and Fred J. Evans. Essex, England: C.W. Daniel Co., Ltd., 1989.

CREDITS

Thanks to the following individuals:

Harry Langdon, photographer (front and back cover, and pages 2 and 7).

Aloma Ichinose, photographer (pages 6, 16, 17, 18, 20, 21, 22, 60, 71, 78, 93, and 102).

Bill Williams, photographer (page 120).

Bill Cuffari, art director (front and back cover; illustrations on pages 14 and 42).

Eric B, art director (illustration on page 119).

James Reva, for fashion design and set decoration.

Trish Garland, Pilates instructor, for body positioning and visual body language.

Robert Ramos, hairstylist (front and back cover).

Aurora Mari, hairstylist (page 120).

Allessandro La Piana, hairstylist (page 7).

Sascha Waugh, makeup artist (front and back cover).

Wayne Massarelli, makeup artist (pages 3 and 6).

David Ditmar, makeup artist (page 7).

Natalie Roux, research and development manager at Rachel Perry, Inc., for special research assistance in sourcing and accessing technical and scientific data.

Melinda Rubin, for special assistance in sourcing out and accessing all aspects of information and data pertinent and vital for thorough coverage of all subject matter from A to Z.

Monica Selanikio, hairstylist, for all-around assistance in coordination of photo sessions.

Brian C. Keller, Ph.D., clinical pharmacologist, investigative dermatologist, and research chemist, for consultations and data on liposome technology and cosmeceutical research.

Peter Stone, D.D.S., assistant professor of clinical dentistry at the University of Southern California School of Dentistry, for consultation on dentistry and its relationship to the visual effect on facial muscular structure and aging.

Timothy Campbell, D.C., for consultation on neuromusculoskeletal relationships.

Bill Landrum, Pilates instructor and choreographer, for consultation and instruction on total muscular regeneration and physical integration.

Stephen Lake, M.D., board-certified plastic and reconstructive surgeon, for consultation on facial exercises and other documented methods of skin and facial rejuvenation.

Uzzi Reiss, M.D., obstetrician/gynecologist, for constulation on hormonal effects on facial aging and data on the adrenal hormone DHEA.

Robert W. Eitches, M.D., board-certified allergist/immunologist, for consultation and data on allergy-related effects causing facial swelling.

George Lieberman, cosmetic research chemist, for consultation on natural skin care formulations.

Mark Blumenthal, president of the American Botanical Society, for massive amounts of data on the benefits of using botanicals, herbs, flora, and fauna in skin care products.

Randy Hayes, president of the Rainforest Action Network, for data on accessing and on the benefits of using sustainably harvested rainforest botanicals in skin care products. I extend to him special recognition for all his hard work and dedication to preserving these precious forests and their residents.

Michael Bishop, research chemist, for consultation and data on hyaluronic acid and skin hydration plus data on anticellulite alternative natural ingredients.

Colin Greene, writer, for literary assistance, copywriting, and photographic and technical advice on all aspects of the manuscript.

And very special thanks to "Paco Perry," my cat and feline son, for his leadership on animal rights, his inspiration, and his very willing and enthusiastic participation in posing for the back cover photo. (Definitely an example of being forever young and beautiful.) "Meow!"

INDEX

Page numbers followed by *(f)* indicate figures; those followed by *(t)*, tables.